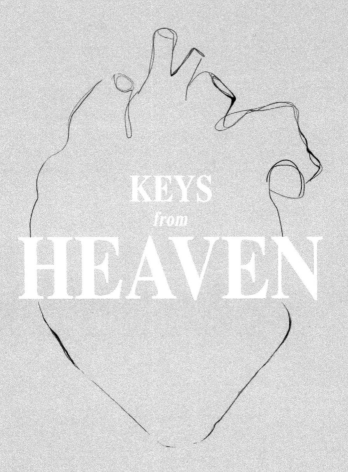

KEYS
from
HEAVEN

KEYS FROM HEAVEN

www.vendelaraquel.com

@vendelaraquel

Copyediting services by Kristen Defevers
Proofreading services by Joanna Kneller
Illustration and graphic design by NormaJean Hill

ISBN: 978-0-578-38456-6

This book is dedicated to the memory of
my beloved father, Al Aguayo.

Dear Dad, thank you for twenty-three years of unconditional
love—the sweetest, purest love. I pray the Lord blesses this
earth with more fathers like Al.

This book is also dedicated to single mothers and orphans.
There is nothing more honorable in God's eyes than looking after
women and children, the fatherless. May God continue to send His
angels to guide, protect, and bless them. May they be filled with life
and love from above as they journey throughout
this earth.

Lastly, this book is dedicated to my Father in heaven. Lord, You
have brought all that is good and worthy of praise into my life. You
have filled me. You believed in me and held me when I was the most
broken. You speak to the depths of my soul, and You are always
there. May more of Your children everywhere experience Your love
and walk in Your freedom. My God, may these writings bless people
and lead them to You. Thank You, Lord, for creating us in Your
image and empowering us to do all things through You. I pray for
the impossible everywhere—the impossible tracing Your fragrance
of wisdom and knowledge.

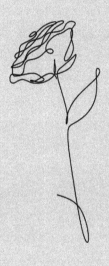

INTRODUCTION

This book is filled with keys from above. Keys that I hope will unlock truth in your everyday life as you sit with it. Truth that empowers you to invite God's Spirit in. Keys that make it simple to choose God each day.

Having God is like having keys to the universe. His Spirit drops the keys in your lap, and it takes faith to pick up each key and unlock the door. It sounds simple, but it takes so much will and power to pick up the keys and use them in your daily life. Keys from our Creator are more powerful than anything else. He is the Alpha and the Omega; He is the beginning and the end. He knows and sees it all, and His keys are better than any promotion, training, practical guidance, inheritance, or opportunity this world can give you.

I had a vision that this book acted as blankets—blankets of God's love. Then God poured down His messengers, and angels laced the sky, delivering blankets to the homes of people everywhere. Freely passed out to all. God is the One Who provides true warmth to your heart, but I pray this book blesses you with His comfort from above and helps you experience His warmth and love—even if it's for just a moment. These writings came to me in the midst of my deepest mourning and pain, the suffering of loss. The pain is what enabled me to write each morning, 378 devotionals over the course of two years. These writings mark the loss of my father and the love God offers when we invite Him into our hurt and pain.

I pray this book provides a display of God's Spirit and fills your life with truth. May we live to experience the sound of heaven touching earth in the hearts and minds of believers everywhere. May chains be broken, and may people walk in freedom and strength that come from above. May we experience God's kingdom here, filled with justice and beauty.

Please find a quiet place and invite God in. In the morning, afternoon, or at night, find your protected time, create the space, and sit with the Divine. With each devotional entry in the pages that follow, you will not only find a key but also a personal reflection, prayer, and Bible verse to help guide your quiet time with God.

So grab your cup of tea and come sit with me.

MEMORIAL OF AL AGUAYO
NAPA, CA

Letter I Read at His Funeral

Love is the most powerful force on this earth. My dad loved being a father and a grandfather. That stemmed from his love for his children. I have never been hugged, kissed, or snuggled more by anyone in my life than my dad. As his daughter, it was nearly impossible to disappoint him—or so he made me feel. My dad could never stay mad at anyone really, but especially me. All I would have to do is wrap my arms around him and smile and he would giggle. My dad was a big teddy bear. Reflecting on all of our memories together, it is the little things I am most grateful for. I now realize the importance of being present for the simple moments because they are filled with so much joy. Dad, I am grateful for our walks along the water in Emeryville and along Fourth Street in Berkeley, our FaceTimes where I tell you at least three times to hit the RED button, and all the mornings where you would run out at 5 a.m. and bring back enough coffee and bagels to Mom's to feed over thirty people. I am grateful for our snuggles while watching the Warriors and our long days at the movie theaters, you picking me up from the Oakland airport and us grabbing Zachary's pizza after, sitting outside of restaurants listening to live music while people watching and eating.

Dad, my heart aches because I thought I'd have you for longer. I never considered what my life would look like without you and now that is a reality I must face. That is where the majority of my hurt stems from, but I am so thankful to have known you and to have had you for as long as I did.

Fathers, look at your daughters as if they can do no wrong. Show them that you desire to spend quality time with them by your actions, that anything they dream of they can have, that they are intelligent and beautiful beyond belief, and that you will always be there to support them. I had this for twenty-three years and I'm beyond blessed because it has shaped who I am, allowed me to accomplish so much, and brought healing to myself and others. I received more love and attention from my dad than some children receive in a lifetime, and I am forever grateful. So much of my strength and confidence stems from the love I received from my father.

Dad, one of the greatest gifts you have left me with is my faith. Any hardship I've ever experienced, same with my brother and mother, we have always had our faith and relationship with God to get us through. That is exactly what this journey of life will be without you, leaning not on our own understandings, but the ways of God. Dad, you taught me from a young age that my faith will always be there; God will always be there.

My friends and family, I encourage you all to pursue this beautiful thing, because it will strengthen you far beyond belief, comfort you in all your days, and give you a clear lens, so that even when pain and heartbreak strike, you can be hopeful, courageous, and find peace.

God, the healing You bring is not of this world, it is incomparable to anything. It is abundant and never runs out.

Dad, you will never be forgotten; there is no one like you. My children will know all about you and so will their children. My heart is at peace knowing you are now in heaven with God. I have so many blessings and having you as a father is by far the greatest. I know that myself, and my family, will be more than okay.

Dad, my promise to you is to love more. Your love lives in me and will be passed on to others. Friends and family, please love the people in your life for everything they are and forget about everything they are not. Dad, thank you. You are so loved and now in a place where all your suffering is over.

I found out on November 22 of 2018, Thanksgiving Day, that my father had passed due to heart failure. Little did I know what was to come after his passing. The suffering, the truth, the freedom, the beauty.

SIX MONTHS

LATER ...

MAY

ABOVE

Above flows an abundance of wisdom, power,
guidance, and pure grace.

Without encouragement and love from God above, I would
have surrendered to my circumstances and the thoughts and
opinions of others.

Put simply, a relationship with your Creator
transforms everything for the
better in your life.

Dear God, I ask that more eyes be opened to your wisdom,
power, guidance, and grace today. Please transform our hearts so
we can move in the direction You have called. Break chains of
fear, anxiety, depression, and anger. May the darkness flee,
and may we hear the sound of chains breaking everywhere.
Fill hearts with love and minds with thoughts from
ABOVE.

Do not be conformed to this world, but be transformed by the renewal of
your mind, that by testing you may discern what is the will of God what
is good and acceptable and perfect.

Romans 12:2 ESV

FIRE

The only person who is at rest has achieved it through
conflict. The mighty peace born of conflict is purified.
Conflict births perspective.

Giving your suffering to God results in
confidence, safety, and peace.

Dear God, time and time again, You have brought me through
the fire. Time and time again, I see how pain pain pain marks my
gain. Help me, Lord, see the place of abundance in the midst of my
pain. It runs, it cuts, it shuts, and it transforms me into something
new. So what is it I cannot do . . . with You? Today
I pray to lay down my old flames to pick up your new
FIRE.

We went through fire and water, but you brought us to
a place of abundance.

Psalm 66:12 NIV

FAITH

When I am broken and hurting, it doesn't feel like
discipline . . . the way I crave You.

It is the discipline of faith that brings
knowledge from God that would
otherwise be impossible.

Faith ~ conviction of things not seen
Faith ~ assurance of things hoped for
Faith ~ complete confidence in someone or something

When you make your request to God it's really
hard to wait, but the key is to keep believing.
Allow your faith to bring you hope and joy
while you wait. This is a muscle;
you must grow in praise and discipline.

Dear God, please grow my faith so I can have conviction,
assurance, and complete confidence in Your will for me,
which is far beyond my wildest dreams! Father,
I pray for greater
FAITH.

Now faith is confidence in what we hope for
and assurance about what we do not see.

Hebrews 11:1 NIV

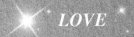 *LOVE*

Suffering produces perseverance, which leads to
learned obedience.

There is glory in our sufferings because
they lead to good character, hope,
and God's love.

God's Love = Agape Love

Agape love is the highest form of love, which is perfect,
unconditional, sacrificial, and pure.

God = Love

Dear Lord, You have brought me through the fire, and
through my sufferings I have grown to know You more
intimately. Because of this, I exist in Your
LOVE.

Love is patient, love is kind. It does not envy, it does not boast, it is not proud.
It does not dishonor others, it is not self-seeking, it is not easily angered, it
keeps no record of wrongs. Love does not delight in evil but rejoices with the
truth. It always protects, always trusts, always hopes, always perseveres.
Love never fails.

1 Corinthians 13:4-8 NIV

OBEDIENCE

When you believe God has your best interest in mind, and that He's all-powerful and all-knowing, you know that your best bet is to trust fully in Him. When you are able to do that, He takes all your anxiety and replaces it with peace and joy.

Obedience is the fruit of faith.

Dear God, I pray for Your will and Your will only. Not because I know Your will, but because I know Your love, and it's oh so sweet and always does right by me. Thank You for all You have done for me. Help me give my life to You. Direct my steps and lace each one with obedience to You Who leads me to my dreams and steadies my heartbeat. Your presence is full of pleasures and fullness of joy. You keep me forevermore. May I learn to move in Your *OBEDIENCE*.

You will show me the path of life; In Your presence is fullness of joy; At Your right hand are pleasures forevermore.

Psalm 16:11 NKJV

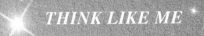

THINK LIKE ME

God's ways are so different compared to the ways of this world.
Oftentimes the way He sees situations and people is the opposite
of how we are taught to see them.

Whenever you are confused or genuinely
don't know the truth, allow God's
words to guide you.

Dear God, help me to think and see like You. Please Lord,
teach me to view people and situations like You, with a
view from above. I no longer want to
THINK LIKE ME.

Finally, brothers and sisters, whatever is true, whatever is noble, whatever is
right, whatever is pure, whatever is lovely, whatever is admirable—if
anything is excellent or praiseworthy—think about such things.

Philippians 4:8 NIV

BELIEVE IT'S TAKEN CARE OF

Sometimes I pray and pray about the same thing, and
I feel like God doesn't deliver. Two keys to keep in mind:

When you send your requests up, release
them and believe they're taken care of.

What's for you will not miss you.

God wants us to believe it's taken care of because He is always in
control, even when it doesn't feel like it. When we believe it's taken
care of, we can have rest. The truth is there are other spiritual forces
that come into play. God is all-powerful, but there is just sooo much
that happens in the spiritual realm that affects our world and truly
surpasses our understanding.

Secondly, what God has for you will not miss you because
God has a way of working everything out for the **GOOD** of His
people. He loves us all so much. Sometimes when you wait longer
for that thing you have been praying about, when it finally does
happen, it is accompanied by new blessings much greater than you
could have imagined.

Dear Lord, if You said it, I believe it. Help me hold close to
Your promises and Word; make it so I
BELIEVE IT'S TAKEN CARE OF.

To the angel of the church in Philadelphia write: These are the words of Him
who is holy and true, who holds the key of David. What He opens no one
can shut, and what He shuts no one can open.

Revelation 3:7 NIV

TALK TO ME

I forget how easily accessible God is. I go through my day-to-day, stressing about silly things, oftentimes feeling overwhelmed by thoughts ❀ and things that may or may not take place in the future.

Be still.

Being still has helped me fight thoughts that do not feed me and helped me learn how to wait on Him. Knowing that there is no such thing as wasted time is key to your peace. God uses it **ALL**. He is never late and knows all your thoughts, desires, and fears. There's nothing He doesn't know about you. He sees you. So, as you quiet yourself, openly bring your thoughts to Him. Not only will it bring you strength, but clarity as well. He's always there.

Dear God, help me be still today. Just long enough so I can hear from You. 🤍
Please Lord,
TALK TO ME.

Be of good courage, and he shall strengthen your heart, all ye that hope in the LORD.

Psalm 31:24 KJV

I STRENGTHEN YOU

God is love.

Love gives you strength.

In any close relationship, listening and loving are key actions. God wants us to listen to His voice and love Him. Not because He needs it, but because He wants to see us prosper.

How do we listen and hear from God?

You listen and sometimes hear from God through His Spirit and with His words. Like any loving relationship, you have to make time for the other person. The more you are able to do that with God, the more clearly you can hear from Him.

Start off small; He will take whatever you give and multiply it! Then you'll reach a point where that is all you want because you start to see all the **POWER** from above fill your life and direct your steps.

Dear Lord, help me make more time for You. Please help me create a space that welcomes You in, even when I don't desire or want to. Please create in me a thirst for You so I can be strong. I know it's Your love that strengthens me. Not I, never could *I STRENGTHEN YOU.*

Trust in him at all times, you people; pour out
your hearts to him, for God is our refuge.

Psalm 62:8 NIV

I AM HERE

God is meticulous. We are like His canvas, and He is the artist. He has the power to paint the most beautiful and highest versions of ourselves if we permit.

One way of allowing Him to transform and create something beautiful in us is by handing over our pain to Him. Life is full of training, and God is doing things in us we do not always understand—this is why He asks us to trust Him in all things.

Refuse to allow your mind to stress about all that is wrong, and watch God move. He is in the middle of your pain, and the more you hand over to Him, the better He can **CREATE** with it.

Give God your pain, and He will
mark your gain.

Dear God, please help me hand my pain over to You. Help me surrender to the pain, help me give my sufferings to You. Do what only You can do. Today, now I ask that You meet me in my pain and transform me into something new. I will wait for You. I will rise early and seek You. Please come;
I AM HERE!

Ask, and it will be given to you; seek, and you will
find; knock, and it will be opened to you.

Matthew 7:7 NKJV

I BREATHE LIFE

Power: We can do anything we put our minds to; we heal, we protect, we overcome, and we lift others up.

Love: We have compassion for those around us, we are quick to forgive, we sacrifice, we know our lives have great value and beautiful plans.

Self-Discipline: Our ways are not always of this world but from the One above. We aim to do what is best according to God so we may be strengthened for all the blessings in our lives and the ones to come.

God breathes life back into us.

The fruits that stem from above are life-giving and fill you with power, love, and self-discipline, growing you in the image of God. Basically, you have permission to do what is **BEST** for you. You can be strong and confident in God, and your life will begin to inspire others and produce fruit.

Dear Lord, today I ask You to breathe life into me. Into all I love, my friends, family, and coworkers. I pray for more of Your breath in my lungs so I can be all You designed me to be! It's You, Your Spirit in me, that makes it so

I BREATHE LIFE!

For God did not give us a spirit of timidity but one of power, love, and self-discipline.

2 Timothy 1:7 ISV

LIGHT THE WORLD

God's love is enough. It's enough for you, for me, for everyone.
The key is allowing Him to take the lead.

He's always there and always present, sometimes it just takes time
to learn the way He communicates. When His ways are first in your
life, you can light 🕯 any and every situation! He equips you with
power and fills you so **YOU** can.

His ways work; they bring relief.

Just ask, and maybe set aside a little quality time, and you'll
start to see the light fill your life and those around you. 🤍

He who is in you is greater than he who is in the world.

1 John 4:4 NKJV

God's love equals a vibrant life filled with joy and purpose. You
can let go and allow Him to direct your steps. The great news is that
anytime we need assurance, He is always there, waiting for us to
draw near. We may fail, but whatever God takes and holds in His
hand, He accomplishes.

Dear Father, You light my life time and time again. I pray
for more of Your light to shine in this world. I ask that You help
me be the light; I want to see the darkness flee! I want to see the
enemy run and relief brought to Your people! Father, it is
You Who lights my world, and only You can
LIGHT THE WORLD.

Delight yourself in the LORD, and he will give you the desires of your heart.

Psalm 37:4 ESV

I AM ENOUGH

God has unlimited resources. His Spirit is with everyone who asks, and His Spirit is always ready to guide; it is sufficient.

Take life one step at a time. Sometimes getting through the day is a victory. Take life moment by moment and remember, you can always call on God's Spirit. He is always there.

Stay in communication with God. He is available any time of the day and loves to listen to our every prayer.

Today I celebrated twenty-four years of life, and one thing I wish I would have done sooner is ask God to send me His Spirit to guide me in all areas of my life. The Spirit of God is enchanted and the greatest resource we have on earth.

Dear Lord, teach me of Your fullness. When I lack, send Your Spirit to fill me with truth. I know with You, I am enough. You are enough for me, oh please just teach me. Teach me to truly believe and embody this as I navigate this world, which at times feels so far from You. Father, with Your Spirit I am empowered to do all You would like me to do;

I AM ENOUGH.

And I will ask the Father, and he will give you another advocate
to help you and be with you forever—the Spirit of truth.

John 14:16-17 NIV

MY TIME

Do not get discouraged, My dear. Sometimes it's the least expected key that opens the door

God's plans are firm and forever. They are to bless you beyond belief. In my life, when a door closes I **REALLY** want to walk through, in time, He opens another. It is always much better and far beyond anything I could have thought for myself.

We must prepare to wait on God's timing; it's precise and it's not for us to know, but to wait and trust.

Allow your waiting seasons to lead you to God.

Of course, you will feel discouraged at times, but you must know that God requires us to wait; it's part of the process. The good news is if it's from above you will not be disappointed, and it will be well worth the wait. Allow your problems to lead you to God. The pleasure in handing your misfortunes over to Him is they can act as reminders to seek God.

Dear Lord, as I grow closer to You in the waiting, bless me with rest and clothe me in Your truth so I can pick up the key that is only from You! May I learn to wait for all things to happen on Your time, not *MY TIME*.

Come to me, all you who are weary and burdened, and I will give you rest. Take my yoke upon you and learn from me, for I am gentle and humble in heart, and you will find rest for your souls.

Matthew 11:28-29 NIV

HOLD ON

There is much to balance in life, so when you feel off, ungrateful, or indifferent (lacking color or zest for life), just hold on to God.

God is our hiding place from the weight of the world 🌐 and while you are in that space just thank Him.

Remove yourself from other people for just a few minutes, find a quiet place, close your eyes, breathe, and ask for peace of mind . . . whatever you need in the moment. Cultivating this habit gives you confidence to tackle the day because you will feel fed emotionally.

Dear Lord, help me hold on to You. I cling to You when I am sad, and You always have the right remedy for me. Oh please, speak to me! I need to hear from You. Please speak to me, because it's only You Who sees me. My heart, soul, and all that troubles me. Hold on to me; please never let go. I always want to *HOLD ON*.

You are my hiding place; you will protect me from trouble and surround me with songs of deliverance.

Psalm 32:7 NIV

IT'S OKAY

There is **SO** much uncertainty in life. So many things are out of our control. I find comfort knowing that God promises to give us peace, and His love will never go anywhere. He is filled with compassion.

Whatever is eating at your peace of mind today, choose to acknowledge it, and act on it . . . but with compassion. ♡

Relationships with people are hard but necessary.
They fill your life with joy.

No matter who disappoints you or what happens in your life, know that you have a God Whose love can't be misplaced. It's full and perfect in every way.

Dear Father, help me remember Your perfect love through the many uncertainties I face. I oftentimes place my identity in my career, hopes, and dreams, but I know all these things will fail me. They are good but not meant to hold the weight I place in them. Only You can hold the weight of my heart. So please, through the uncertainty, remind me that all will be okay because I have You, God the Almighty, forever with me. I have You to always remind me *IT'S OKAY.*

"For the mountains may depart and the hills be removed, but my steadfast love shall not depart from you, and my covenant of peace shall not be removed," says the LORD, who has compassion on you.

Isaiah 54:10 ESV

REST IN ME

I so easily put my worth in my accomplishments or how much I am doing. Restless working gets you nowhere. I say this to you now, and yet I continue to do it, time and time again. Sleepless nights, wasted time, and busyness that leave me feeling empty. It leads to a cycle of desperately wanting to check things off your list, but there will always be another accomplishment bigger than the last that eats away at you. You are left wanting more of something else.

Stop your restless working and listen; wait in silence for your Creator to direct your next steps. Clear out one thing in your day, and replace it with quality time with God. Then you will know what is draining you and what is feeding you, pushing you forward.

The truth is God has more to give than we could ever **WORK** for, simply because He is God . . . the Creator of all things, the Alpha and the Omega, the beginning and the end. He has an exhaustive treasury that never runs out. Lay it at His feet, and God will give you an overflowing cup.

Once you tap into His presence, experience His Spirit, and are comforted by His ways, there is no need to ever rely on anything else. I have experienced this in my life, but my flesh seems to get the best of me at times. However, God's tender nature is not of this world 🌐 and keeps me coming back.

Dear Father, show me what it looks like to find rest in You. Fill my cup, make it overflow, and show me where You'd like it to go! When I rest with You, I know my very next step and can move forward, flying high in the sky, because You are giving me my wings. It's You Who places

REST IN ME.

But those who hope in the LORD will renew their strength. They will soar on wings like eagles; they will run and not grow weary; they will walk and not be faint.

Isaiah 40:31 NIV

THANK ME

So often I go through life rushing. I am working on intentional reflection. When I carve out time and space to reflect, I can better see the blessings in front of me, and I am filled with gratitude. There is so much beauty in my life that I take for granted. There are so many open doors I have walked through that were blessings from above, and yet I am so quick to forget.

There is power in gratitude and praising God for how far His love and protection has brought you.

God is the only One Who can keep us safe, and acknowledging what He has done in your life brings more truth, more beauty, more blessings, and more freedom from others' thoughts or actions towards you that are not whole.

Dear Lord, thank You for all You have done and all You continue to do. Shame on me, I am sorry for my continued lack of gratitude. I might never get it right, but today I choose to see You and where You have brought me. Fear may come knocking tomorrow, but I choose to see You Who keeps me safe and desires nothing but good for me. For it is all You, my author of all that is good, it will always be You I thank. Never can I look and see all You have done through me and
THANK ME.

Fearing any human being is a trap, but confiding in the LORD keeps anyone safe.
Proverbs 29:25 ISV

COME TO ME

If you're like me, your heart gets heavy. Your mind gets heavy. It's almost like there needs to be a reset button. It's easy to try and not feel things, but that's not a healthy outlook to have.
It makes you less human, less aware, and hurts your ability to problem-solve.

The best and most effective reset button for me is prayer. When I talk to God, He gives me simple truths that make everything less heavy and more clear.

Sometimes I feel like I need permission from others to be me, a horrible habit I am working on breaking. But when God communicates with you, it's freeing because He gives you strength so you can be yourself and walk confidently.

Being yourself doesn't mean you're perfect, it just means you are perfect the way He created you.

God gives permission to be anything you desire that is good. Not that you need permission, but this world has a way of making you think differently about yourself.

Dear Lord, wake me each day and lead me to Your truth. Help me pray and meditate with You. Lead me down the path You wish, and bless me with abundance. Abundant freedom, rest, peace, confidence, strength, and truth. Father,
COME TO ME.

This is the confidence we have in approaching God: that
if we ask anything according to his will, he hears us.

1 John 5:14 NIV

I AM IN YOU

Ever since I was a little girl, I've always felt something with me, beside me—something comforting me. As I got older, that feeling faded.

When we are young, we have an innocence about us, maybe because there is so much we have not seen, experienced, or gone through yet. We see the world so differently. When I reflect on my life, my worldview was the strongest and most pure when I was just a little girl. My standards and morals were so much easier to uphold due to my perspective.

When we invite God in, we are protected in the same way a child is. He restores our worldview. 🖤

God is in and with children, but He is also in and with us. The more room you make, the more He dwells in you. Suddenly your perspective shifts back to the purest worldview, back to when you were a child . . . even after all you've gone through and all you've seen.

Dear Jesus, we have yet to meet, but thank You for what You have done for me. I know it was Your Spirit that comforted me when I was just a little girl. I know it was Your Spirit that whispered to me. I pray for a childlike heart, mind, and eyes. May Your Spirit never leave me, let us become one, for I dwell with You,
I AM IN YOU.

But Jesus said, "Let the children come to me. Don't stop them! For the Kingdom of Heaven belongs to those who are like these children."

Matthew 19:14 NLT

I PROTECT

I am a tree that has been cut down more than once, but the growth promotes new life, causing me to rise higher and higher towards the sky, with a heavenly glow warming my insides like the sun. You help me grow and venture to worlds unknown.

This world 🌏 can be hard to navigate. God knows how confused we feel at times, no matter how many times we try or switch up our approach, He knows how difficult this journey of life can be.

Don't be fooled by the way things seem or appear
at a certain point in time. Our view is limited,
but God's is limitless!

He is protecting and leading us on straight paths even when it doesn't feel like it. Sometimes God has to make new wine out of you . . . in the crushing and the pressing He creates something new. 🍇 🍷

When you trust, you don't need to understand.

Dear God, thank You for Your loving hand over my life. I know I don't always choose You, but thank You for always choosing me. Thank You for the mighty protection of the seen and unseen. Oh, please keep me on Your straight path, protect my steps, and teach me the ways of wisdom. May my choices honor You and bring new life and growth to the garden of fruits *I PROTECT.*

I instruct you in the way of wisdom and lead you along straight paths.

Proverbs 4:11 NIV

JUNE

GIVE MORE TO ME

Worry. I worry about my family. I worry about my friends. I worry about people I love. I worry about what doors will open, what doors will close. I worry about the future. I worry about what is out of my control. I worry about what is in my control!

Why do we worry so much? This is not to say that there are not heavy things that cause us stress . . . but worry itself, what does it actually do for you or me?

Worrying does nothing for anyone or any situation.

I am learning to acknowledge worry. The reasons that cause us to worry are fair, but surrendering those worries to God will be the only thing that brings peace.

Why should we give our worry to Him?

God, the Creator of the universe, loves when we give our worries over to Him. The best part is, once we learn to do this, in exchange for the worry, He gives us peace. God made beautiful plans for each person He created, and He alone knows the end result—after all, He is the beginning and the end. There is usually a much deeper meaning behind the things that happen to us in life.

Trust God's ways of bringing about His plans for your life because they are infinitely wise.

Dear Father, show me how to give my worries to You. My God, You painted the sky, carved the moon, and gathered the winds in Your fists. It is You Who instructs me, asking that I not be anxious about anything. So please, show me how to do this! I lift my worries up to You today and thank You for the peace You will plant in me, preparing me so You can
GIVE MORE TO ME.

Do not be anxious about anything, but in every situation, by prayer and petition, with thanksgiving, present your requests to God.

Philippians 4:6 NIV

TAKE IT TO ME

Sometimes it's hard for me to let go and slow down. God wants me to take it to Him. The truth is that for everything I have brought to God, He then takes it and makes a way forward. Usually, it's a way that I could have never imagined or could have never done on my own.

Sometimes our greatest gain in life may come through our greatest pain. Finding acceptance in this is challenging but powerful. And what's even more powerful is laying it at God's feet.

If God is truly sovereign, then you must know He is there and still in control in times of darkness and chaos. And only He can empower you to turn the darkness into light.

God is our constant companion, and He will
enable you to see His love, truth, beauty,
healing, and light in the midst of your
loss, if you allow Him to.

Do not focus on the loss, circumstance, lie,
or negative narrative in your life that is
weighing you down.

Dear God, I have a very broken heart. I miss my dad every day, but I know, I believe with every ounce of me, that You will use my pain. So, I thank You for today and all the good You desire to give me. It's the plans You whisper to me that give me hope for the future. I know how close You are to my broken heart and the good You desire for me. So today I pray You continue to comfort me

and those who suffer from losses similar to mine. Speak to
the depths of their hearts as You do for me, and whisper
to their hearts and minds,
TAKE IT TO ME.

That is what the Scriptures mean when they say, "No eye has seen,
no ear has heard, and no mind has imagined what God has prepared
for those who love Him."

1 Corinthians 2:9 NLT

June 3, 2019

LAY BY ME

When we lay by God, everything we thought was so urgent seems to take a back seat—and maybe not stress us out as much. The best relief you can find in life comes by stopping and taking a moment or two to lay, and just be with the Creator of the universe.

Your busy schedule, the balance you are trying to find, that thing you have to get done, **WALK AWAY** from it, and lay by God. I close the door, light a candle, make a cup of tea, and breathe. Or I go for a walk and take in the fresh air. Whatever it is I do, it's important that my time is quiet and untouched, creating a space to pray and wait for His presence, His Spirit to enter.

The Lord will refresh your soul.

Dear Father, thank You for showing me what it looks like to create space for You in my life. I have keys to unlocking peace. I now have habits that promote peace! Time with You, Your gentle Spirit, will be enough to get me through. Oh, You Who refreshes my soul, You are too good to me. I don't understand, but grateful I am. Please continue to
LAY BY ME.

The LORD is my shepherd, I lack nothing. He makes me lie down in green pastures, he leads me beside quiet waters, he refreshes my soul.

Psalm 23:1-3 NIV

✦ *LOVE ME* ·

I have found that when I focus on loving God more, I am a better friend, aunt, daughter, coworker, and all-around person. I sometimes get overwhelmed with balancing relationships in my life, and as a result, I pull away from people because I feel spread thin and am falling short with the people I care for.

When I asked God how I can better love Him, He gave me these three keys:

Love people, but especially those in your life who need it the most.

Quality time with Me.

I try and fill my mornings with quiet time, just me, God, and my morning matcha, of course! Or I go for evening sunset walks.

Praise Me and when people ask, be truthful, sweet Vendy.

I try to give answers that I feel speak to people, so in the past I have crafted something that might have left God out of the equation. I know now that when you are truthful in sharing where God's love has brought you and all He has done, it's better. Not because it's true for everyone but chances are, if He has moved in my life like this, He's probably doing it all around the world 🌍 for **SOOOOOO** many people!

Dear God, thank You for loving me. Thank You for showing me how to love. Thank You for all the love I have in my life, from family and close friends. Help me keep You first so I can love more fully. Oh, please don't ever stop, always *LOVE ME.*

Beloved, let us love one another, for love is from God, and whoever loves has been born of God and knows God. Anyone who does not love does not know God, because God is love.

1 John 4:7-8 ESV

KEEP GOING

There is no need to put limits or boundaries on our relationship
with God. He will never take advantage, He will never fail you,
and He will never leave you. Our Creator wants us to be confident,
especially in this! We were not created to have timid spirits,
and when we know God's heart and how He views us, we are
empowered to keep going. We are fueled and can keep striving after
that desire that was placed in us by God.

God has a limitless mind.

We should strive to see things through His mindset. Just do
the things that are in your power and God will do the rest!

Don't make yourself small
for others . . . not everyone
wants to see you thrive.

God's heart for us is to see us thrive and walk in our true identity.
This is powerful because we live in a world with narratives designed
to tear us down and separate us from His love.

The Spirit that enabled people to change the world 🌍 throughout
history is the same Spirit that is freely available to us today. Practice
faith, choose hope, act in love, and know all things are
possible 🤍 with God.

Dear Lord, I love how close I am growing to You. I can hear
You, and Your truth is cutting through lies that live in my mind.
Oh, God, thank You. Because of You, chains are breaking,
limits are disappearing, and I am able to
KEEP GOING.

There is surely a future hope for you, and your hope will not be cut off.

Proverbs 23:18 NIV

I KNOW YOUR HEART

Sometimes when I pray, I talk to God as if He does not already
know my every thought.

The truth is that He knows everything about us: our
deepest thoughts, every desire, and even the
emotions we will encounter tomorrow.

So instead of praying about all that was on my mind today,
I asked God to tell me about my heart. He said I have
faith, I am strong, not always the most logical, and my
heart is tender.

Sometimes when you are confused about what is next, or life itself,
instead of sending requests up, just ask God to share His point
of view with you. He knows every prayer in our hearts, and it's
insightful to hear the Lord's take on things.

Dear God, it's You Who knows my heart. It's You Who wonderfully
created me. Teach me how You'd like me to see things. You Who are
familiar with my ways, free me from my irrational ways and show
me how to be more like You because You are all that is good.
I KNOW YOUR HEART.

You know when I sit and when I rise; you perceive my thoughts from afar.
You discern my going out and my lying down; you are familiar
with all my ways. Before a word is on my tongue
You, LORD, know it completely.

Psalm 139:2-4 NIV

I GOT YOU

With every turn in the road, you can find something wrong and allow it to rob you of your peace of mind. It could even be a good thing, a blessing, but you just don't know what the right move is, and so you stress about making the right decision. Point being, instead of being grateful or reflective of certain milestones in our lives, we get hung up and worry. And as a result, we are quick to forget past blessings or the ways things have worked out.

Lifting your heart to God in a moment of faith can quickly change your view of the circumstance you are in. He makes a way when there is no way. He is always in control even when it doesn't feel like it.

It's a moment-by-moment, day-by-day struggle to hand things over to God, but the more you can practice doing it, the more joy you will have; your worry will fade. The Creator of all is in control. He is good, and when you surrender to His plan for your life, you are choosing the best possible plan.

Dear God, grateful I am for how tight You hold me. Close to You I now dwell, and because of this I can more easily give You my worries and cares. It's You Who comforts my broken heart, it's You Who holds me and rocks me to sleep. It's You Who greets me in the morning. You, my Lord, sustain me, and forever I will serve You. My life is now Yours,
I GOT YOU.

Cast your cares on the LORD and he will sustain you; he will never let the righteous be shaken.

Psalm 55:22 NIV

BE WITH ME

I rush a lot—something I wish I did not do. When you are rushing from one thing to the next, you are missing simple, beautiful truths and moments in life.

God helps me see the things I overlook each day when I take time to be with Him. This morning He told me how He wants me to love, and it's the same way He has loved me . . . without boundaries. Sometimes I put walls up and create structure for how I love someone. You do this, I do that—and I call it love. But to care for another person without boundaries is powerful; it takes trust and forgiveness.

When you care for people in your life without keeping track of the rights or wrongs, your love is purified.

Love is a verb, not a noun. When we love without boundaries, we heal each other. You also demonstrate trust in God by doing right by people, which makes our Creator smile.

Dear God, today I pray for more of Your love to fill the spaces and places that need it most. I know when I love without boundaries it is not because I will not get hurt, I most likely will, but it's because I trust in You and Your ways, which will never lead me astray. Love is the only thing in my life that has been able to cast out fear. Lord, I ask more love to be spread from above as we learn to sit with You. My best days are the days I choose to sit with You, so please, Lord, always *BE WITH ME.*

Trust in the LORD and do good; dwell in the land and enjoy safe pasture.

Psalm 37:3 NIV

EVERY STEP

Memories sweeten life. It's a beautiful thing to sit and reflect.
To remember past times in your life. Sometimes I catch myself
drifting, and I am reminded that God is constantly moving forward,
and He is consistently pushing us forward as well. It can be scary to
take steps in life, but keep moving forward, always.

God is with us through the good and the bad. If we want,
He promises to direct our steps, one at a time.

There is much comfort in this because, even if you don't understand
your now, you can find hope knowing that all the pieces in your life
will come together for the good because of the kind Creator Who is
in control. All you have to do is hold on to His ways, allowing love
and truth to lead the way; everything else will fall into place.

Sometimes that next step is uncomfortable and painful, but the
more you are able to move forward with a faith perspective
in life, the more full your life will be.

Dear God, establish my every step. I pray for Your will to be
done on earth as it is in heaven for my life and the lives of all
Your people. My Lord, help me keep going. Plant my each step
with hope and peace. Some days more than others, I think of my
loss, my sweet father, and the way my life was before, but I know
You will take good care of me. You will, my sweet God, bless me
with more beautiful memories, people, and a deep love.
For it is You Who protects my
EVERY STEP.

In their hearts humans plan their course, but the LORD establishes their steps.

Proverbs 16:9 NIV

SEE LIKE ME

Sometimes we get in our own heads. We create a story and stand in offense, but when we ask God to help us see like Him, grace enters and we are able to see things differently. Then comes the peace.

God helps us to see like Him so we can have grace, a sound mind, and confidence moving forward.

Dear Lord, in my weakness I have seen Your moves best. Only You can do what You have done for me in my weakness. When I experience pain, You help me choose love. When I am lost, You show me the way. When I am lonely, You draw even closer. When I am broken, You give me wings. When I am blind, You open my eyes. When I bend a knee to fear, Your love lifts me. I pray for more people to invite You in, so we may have more open eyes that see like You. No longer do I care to *SEE LIKE ME.*

But he said to me, "My grace is sufficient for you,
for my power is made perfect in weakness."

2 Corinthians 12:9 NIV

✦ *LOOK TO ME* ✦

God is not a man, so he does not lie. He is not human, so he does not change his mind.
Has he ever spoken and failed to act? Has he ever promised and not carried it through?

Numbers 23:19 NLT

Some of the greatest lessons of life are birthed from pain. When
I experienced a great loss, I had to learn, and still am learning, how
to have joy again. I just didn't feel safe in this world 🌍 , but God
was able to reach me in my brokenness and comfort me so much that
I am able to look back at my loss and see it in a new light.
Grateful I now am for it even.

Weary, tender heart, you must not be discouraged
but be glad of the sorrows that sow
because from them virtues flow that grow,
allowing you to dance in the rain,
freeing you from the shame.
With each sunset and rising moon, the time will pass
and you will one day see it was He Who got you through,
planted a garden and prepared a harvest fit for a queen.
Oh weary, tender heart you are destined for
mighty, mighty things!

In the midst of your stress, pain, change, and the
unknown, just focus on God.

Dear Lord, You have a way of working everything out for our
good. So, when I start to worry about things, help me look to You.
It is You Who looks after me, watching my every move, and as a
result, I pray others may see You in me when they
LOOK TO ME!

Why are you in despair, my soul? Why are you disturbed within me? Hope
in God, for once again I will praise him, since his presence saves me.

Psalm 42:5 ISV

STOP

Stop so you can tune out others' opinions of you
Stop so you can take things in and be grateful
Stop so you can have freedom
from the weight in your life
Stop so you can love yourself
Stop so you can listen
Stop so you can have freedom
Stop so you can push the world out

Our Creator sees things differently and calls His people to freedom. Freedom to choose but also freedom to be who we are without caring what people think we should be like based on our age, education, career, past, or whatever standards people use to measure others.

Stop so you can have tranquility with your thoughts. When you stop, you give your mind time to recharge. When you stop, you can invite God's Spirit in.

Dear Father, lies fill Your people's minds. Please God, I pray against the attacks of the enemy. I want to see him flee, I want to see an end to his pain-filled ways and trickery. My sweet Lord, help us stop long enough to invite You in. Please, we invite Your Spirit in to dwell close. My God, thank You for our mornings and meditations. Oh, how much they help me with my thoughts. Thank You for helping me slow down and
STOP.

Do you not know that you are God's temple and that
God's Spirit dwells in you?

1 Corinthians 3:16 ESV

IT'S DONE

Our Creator dominates over the impossible. No matter your circumstance, He can make the impossible possible. I have seen and experienced this in my life many times. It's almost like with God things are **SOOO** much easier. I tend to struggle with faith, but it is so key to experiencing God move. It's hard to cultivate, but it's the one ingredient that is in our control, and He only requires a little of it.

When we feed our faith, our fears starve. If you are not doing something because of fear, then you should do that thing because fear doesn't come from God; to do something that scares you takes faith!

When you act in faith, it forces you to let go, and it allows God to do His thing.

The Creator of the universe is much more powerful than we are. So really, what seems riskier is actually the safest route you can go.

Faith honors God, and God delights in our faith.

With faith . . . it's done.

Dear Father, You know my every heart's desire. You know some of these dreams, they scare me. You know that some of the things You will call me to do one day will take mighty faith, so show me how to grow it. Help me believe and trust not all I see,

but You. Father, I know that faith is all it takes! With faith,
even in the midst of others' disbelief, Your will,
IT'S DONE.

This is why the promise is by faith, so that it may be according
to grace, to guarantee it to all the descendants.

Romans 4:16 CSB

I HOLD YOU

The loss of my dad broke me. I have always been a joyful person, filled and bubbling over with life, but this was the first time in my life where the lights went completely out. The pain was visible in my eyes; I have never felt so broken before. The suffering cut deep, and it was unlike anything I had ever experienced.

Today is an emotional day for me, but also one I am grateful for. I am grateful for the beautiful twenty-three years I had with the most loving father. Although his body is no longer with me on earth 🌍 , God has moved in and replaced much of his absence.

Our Creator holds broken people and things together. If He were not doing so, they would fall apart because that's what broken things do—they crumble into pieces.

You are not the only one who has ever felt broken. Allow the pain you experience to give life to someone else.

Dear Lord, my sweet One Who keeps me. Thank You for rebuilding me. You keep us whole in our brokenness. You fill our weakness with Your strength. You save each tear and sprinkle it over someone else's garden to give them strength and help them grow. Thank You, my God, for the precious jewels You have bestowed in me. May You always hold me and may always *I HOLD YOU.*

O storm-battered city, troubled and desolate! I will rebuild you with precious jewels and make your foundations from lapis lazuli.

Isaiah 54:11 NLT

✦ *CHOOSE ME* ✦

When you choose God, you open your life to infinite possibilities.
He is always choosing us, but we do not always choose Him.

I have wasted a lot of energy not choosing God. When I quiet
my spirit and I am open to whatever He has for me, I hear Him
better, and it makes it easier for me to choose God because I can
better understand His ways.

Give yourself time to choose so you can act out of
a space filled with faith.

Dear soul be still.
The willing and waiting Spirit is ready to heal.

Dear soul be still.
The willing and waiting Spirit is ready to fill.

Dear soul be still.
The willing and waiting Spirit is ready for the thrill!

Dear Lord, my broken heart and torched soul are finally ready to be
still. It took twenty-three years to shake, quiet, and wake my kind
soul, but You are never a day late! I pray to always seek You. May
I always seek You in the morning, seek You in the evening, seek
You more than I seek any desire or dream I crave. My God, I pray
for more souls to choose You. Oh, Father, I just hope, I ask, that
when I get to the gates, I pray, I pray You
CHOOSE ME.

The LORD is good to those who wait for Him, To the soul who seeks Him.

Lamentations 3:25 NKJV

I HAVE BEST

We can conquer anything that sets us back in life. However, two things must take place to overcome. First, you must believe you can overcome through hope or faith. Second, you must surrender to God. If you do not believe it is even possible, then you will never start, and if you never surrender to a higher power, you have not conquered but simply covered! Surrendering to God brings two keys:

Surrender allows the natural process of healing to take place because it opens your hands.

When you truly surrender something, your expectations change—or fade, I should say.

Unmet expectations can cause detours. I know for me, when an expectation is not met, I tell myself, "It's just not meant to be," and I am more likely to give up. The danger in this is when the disappointment is so great, it becomes challenging to get back up.

Know God has the best plan for your life. You want His Plan A because His Plan A for your life is filled with peace, beauty, power, and it's the best possible version. You are protected and living with joy. You conquer all things because you are dwelling with God, living His Plan A.

Pay as little attention to discouragement as possible.

How do we live out Plan A?

We must do our best to do right by others, placing love
and forgiveness first, and be humble and kind, knowing
everything you have been given and blessed with comes
from God's goodness.

Dear Lord, I write to You today knowing that You have a master
plan for my life, and it is Your will I pray to be done. Please Lord,
close the doors that are not from You, and protect me when I grow
weak so I can stay on Your path. Father, I know You have the best
plan. I want to wake up each day knowing I have what
You intended for me, knowing
I HAVE BEST.

He has shown you, O mortal, what is good. And what does the LORD
require of you? To act justly and to love mercy and to walk
humbly with your God.

Micah 6:8 NIV

I MAKE NEW

I am learning that sometimes to be a blessing to someone else means you need to have gone through some sorrow on your end. It's almost like that's the price you pay to have the privilege of comforting others.

While you are being ground into bread to feed others, know that hardships and misfortunes have propelled people throughout history and this world 🌎 to a life of greatness. Pain and challenges shift your perspective and strengthen your soul. And with that, you are made new.

My sweet Vendy, I have saved every tear
in a glass bottle and I will use them to water
seeds that spring to life

Seek Him; more time with God gives you
peace and strength.

Dear Father, thank You for the many tears I have shed. Because my tender heart has journeyed through much, I will be a blessing to others. Lord, our stories of pain mold us into something new and bring glory to You and Your Kingdom when we learn to hand them over to You. When we learn to let You fight our battles. My Lord, use me! Use me, do whatever You have to do to make me new.
Oh, I know my God, through You
I MAKE NEW!

Grain must be ground to make bread.

Isaiah 28:28 NIV

I'M IN CHARGE

If we truly believe God is in charge, we will worry less. But our human minds like things to go the way we **THINK** they should go, and we have a hard time trusting.

Talking and hearing from God is how you will receive the most peace because the Creator of the universe is the most powerful source you could ever tap into.

How do we hear more clearly from God?

Find a quiet place and be still.

Focus all your attention on God in devotion
(even though memories or random
thoughts may pop in).

Cultivate an eagerness to know His will.

Your answer may come through His Scripture, a thought, words, or encouragement from a friend or family member. It may manifest in the form of a closed door or an open door. Either way, when you seek God with your heart and mind, I promise you, He will arrive. Your life will begin to be filled with peace. It just takes strength to wait in silent expectation, because it's the opposite of what the world, our culture, teaches us. This world craves an immediate answer, and although God sometimes delivers immediate answers, dropping keys in your lap, He also does the opposite and requires us to wait on Him.

Dear Lord, I have learned the hard way what it means to wait on You. But now that I have the key, spending time with You, I pray to never turn back to my old ways. I always want to wait on You, because I know what You have, what You do, is far greater than anything I could have worked out on my own. Father, forever be the captain of my ship. With Your Spirit leading the way, how could I go wrong? You protect my steps and send wisdom to guide the way. You give me free will and let me choose between different possible courses of action unhindered. You make it so

I'M IN CHARGE.

Whether you turn to the right or to the left, your ears will hear
a voice behind you, saying, "This is the way; walk in it."

Isaiah 30:21 NIV

I LISTEN

As people, it's important we feel heard. It's hard for me to imagine what God looks like, and when I describe Him, I often give Him human characteristics because that's all I know.

This morning God heard me. He heard every one of my requests because He listens. He may not grant you everything, but He knows what's on your heart and hears it all.

Be thankful for your blessings, but be willing to lay them down. Be willing to release them back to God if need be.

When I lost my dad, it was important for me to focus on all the good I still had. But more importantly, the loss of my dad taught me that **EVERYTHING** I hold on to could be gone tomorrow, so understanding that God will never leave you is where you find true rest and ultimate joy.

Dear Lord, You have let me in and I never want to go back. The veil has been lifted and I can now see! I can see it is You Who takes care of me, loves me tenderly, and hears me. Thank You for all the good in my life, I know it's all from You, and should I lose a love tomorrow or sometime soon, I have comfort and peace knowing I will always still have You. So, help me choose You. Now, God, if You speak, *I LISTEN*.

Therefore, we who have fled to him for refuge can have great confidence as we hold to the hope that lies before us. This hope is a strong and trustworthy anchor for our souls. It leads us through the curtain into God's inner sanctuary.

Hebrews 6:18-19 NLT

✦ *LOVE LIKE ME* ✦

It's easy to be mad at someone, especially when you feel wronged by them. Especially when you don't approve of their decisions. Especially when they have hurt the people you love.

There has been one relationship in my life where instead of leading with love, I consistently led with conflict. The crazy part is, during that season of my life, I thought I was doing the right thing, but looking back, the truth is I was only making matters worse by not leading with love.

I was fighting a very real battle with fire, and it made the flames even bigger, which caused burns that led to scars. This battle was with my sister, who is severely mentally ill. She was making decisions that brought harm to herself, and as a result, she was hurting the people I loved the most: my parents, grandparents, aunts, uncles, and so on. This pained me for many years. I was very mean to my sister—harsh words and a condemning spirit drove me. Unfortunately, I lacked a deeper understanding of the roots that caused much of my sister's turmoil. But it's not about knowing or understanding what someone else goes through, it's about fighting battles with the breastplate of love. Love acts as a shield; it becomes your breastplate.

The best way to fight battles in your life is with love. When you choose to fight your battles with love, you are made blameless and love always wins.

Choose love as a response in all your relationships because love will heal. It doesn't make

everything go away, but it acts as water, slowly
putting out the burning flames that are eating at
the people involved.

When you choose love, not only is it better for your
own mind, heart, and well-being, but you start to
see the different layers and understand why that person
acted the way they did. You will find that nine out of ten
times when a person wrongs you or themselves, it's their
own pain behind it. You can choose to add to it or heal it.

Dear Father, forgive me. I have greatly hurt Your daughter, my
sister, whom I know You love. I have hurt a person who is hurting
so much that she continues to inflict pain upon herself. I promise
to do my best to lead with love. The shame and guilt I have felt
for putting my sister down is something I struggle with. Lord,
I pray to do right by You. I give You my life to fight on behalf
of these suffering souls. Please forgive me. I want to love like You.
And I pray to never repeat the same mistake I have made with my
sister; cultivate in me wisdom and understanding so I can love
new. Redeeming is Your love. Father, make my love cover all
wrongs. Make my love pure like You. Remove the hatred that
stirred up conflict and bring streams of healing that could have
only be from above. Streams of healing taught by the Son.
He is the One who teaches and says,

Sweet V,
LOVE LIKE ME.

Hatred stirs up conflict, but love covers over all wrongs.

Proverbs 10:12 NIV

I'M ALWAYS HERE

Sometimes I get busy and put things first that I don't always want to but feel like I should. Whatever your routine is, you can always invite God in; He is continually watching over us. You can always look up and send a quick "Thank You" or "Help me" or "I miss You" in the midst of whatever you are doing. It doesn't always have to be when you are isolated or alone.

Intimacy with our Creator is enhanced by adversity, but also by refusing to rely on our own understanding.

Friendly Reminder: God is always there and always with you. Just smile to yourself, look up, and say whatever you want to say in your mind and heart. It's a quick message that goes up and suddenly you have a lifeline lifting your spirits.

Dear God, thank You for my matcha as I drive to work this morning. Thank You for the view along Pacific Coast Highway. Thank You for these tunes and thank You for the pain I walk through. If it weren't for the pain, I would have never learned how to trust You. I would have never appreciated the little things the way I do. Father, never leave my side, oh please take me where You'd like me to go! *I'M ALWAYS HERE.*

Trust in and rely confidently on the Lord with all your heart
And do not rely on Your own insight or understanding.

Proverbs 3:5 AMP

I CONTROL THE WIND

Our entire lives will be filled with strong winds—winds that are powerful, winds that can blow us away or knock us down.

God has control over the wind. God has control over these winds, and you have control over whether you get blown away or ask God to help you walk through them.

The forces at play in life that block your progress are at God's command. If you hand over to Him the material designed to stop you, He uses it to empower you. He is a God known for making a way when there is no way. What was meant to destroy you, He uses for your good. Now that is something only God can do.

Accept that there will always be strong, uncontrollable winds in life, but with God, you can learn how to have peace of mind while they are blowing.

We will be robbed of a beautiful life if we focus on all that is wrong—the strong winds.

Choose to see your situation through the lens of God, Who is all-powerful and uses your setbacks as game changers for the better.

Dear God, I now know that when the winds of life blow, when the strong winds knock me down, I need not fear because You have the power to use these winds for my good! Father, with You, Your mighty Spirit that dwells with me, I am unshaken.

Father, I welcome the strong winds, my heart is undaunted because I trust in You. The winds no longer dictate my steps, cause panic, or fill me with distress. Nope. With You Lord, You make it so

I CONTROL THE WIND!

He need not fear a bad report, for his heart
is unshaken, since he trusts in the LORD.

Psalm 112:7 ISV

I ALWAYS ANSWER

Sometimes when I don't know what to do (no matter how big or small), rather than enter into prayer, I call my family, friends, or people I trust and talk it over to process with them. This usually gives me peace in the moment, but it doesn't last. Shortly after I am confused and filled with doubt.

When I go straight to God in prayer, not only does He provide an answer, but also, whatever it is, even if I don't fully understand, He brings me lasting peace. I remind myself I heard from the Creator of the universe. It's all good.

Yesterday I went on a walk and a few things were on my mind concerning a decision I had to make. Instead of calling someone to process my thoughts and seek advice, I waited on God to give me clarity.

Our Creator rarely tells us what to do. He just allows us to see things clearly so we can make a decision that comes from a place of love. That comes from a place of faith and hope. And when you act from that place, the outcome of your life starts to reflect godly qualities of faith, hope, and love.

Dear Father, thank You for meeting me in the middle of my confusion, doubt, and fear. When I don't know which way to go, You steer me clear. You, my dear Lord, are so good to me.

I know I grow impatient; I know I don't always wait on You, but I pray to cultivate this trait. To wait for You. It's You, to You may *I ALWAYS ANSWER.*

This is the confidence we have in approaching God: that if we ask anything according to his will, he hears us. And if we know that He hears us—whatever we ask—we know that we have what we asked of Him.

1 John 5:14-15 NIV

SEE ALL THE POSSIBILITIES

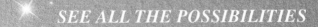

I've always been a dreamer. I've always hoped for the impossible. However, the older I get and the more hardships I face, the more limits enter my mind. I probably do this subconsciously because I think I am protecting myself . . .

A relationship with God allows you to see **ALL** the possibilities in life, so when you are about to walk away, He will suddenly speak to your spirit and say, "Knock just one more time," or "I can make a way; just be still, I go before you."

No matter your circumstance, do not limit your mind. If you pursue a relationship with your Creator, that is the very ground He takes over—your mind. With this shift in perspective, you start to experience outcomes you didn't know were possible simply because you believed. You had hope. You were courageous. Your heart was in the right place. You acted with compassion. You acted with all the other fruits that God blessed your spirit with, so you were able to embody them all.

Dear God, I know I move and act from places of fear, but the closer I grow to You, the more limitless I feel. I just can't help but thank You for this. My Lord, thank You for the shift in perspective and atmosphere You create in my life. I pray more of Your people begin to experience this. I pray, Lord, You bless the dreams of this world. You gave us these dreams for a reason. May our vision be from You as we grow to *SEE ALL THE POSSIBILITIES.*

And to know this love that surpasses knowledge—that you may be filled to the measure of all the fullness of God.

Ephesians 3:19 NIV

✦ *I LOVE YOU* ✦

Love unites. When you encounter a person who loves well, it's usually because they have been shown love. They have been loved on by another human—maybe a parent, friend, partner—or God.

When you have love, you are full and you can give love. When we feel hurt or lonely, we don't always give love to others the way we should.

It's easy to love the people in your life who are good to you, the people you get along with. The challenge is showing love to the person you don't see eye to eye with. The person who maybe hasn't received as much love as you and can be cold or hurtful.

The cold, rude person in your life is the one that needs love the most. If you can just meet them with love every time they are hostile towards you, you will be amazed at the shift in atmosphere. You may even see their heart warm.

I am not saying you should go out of your way for people who are rude or disrespectful towards you, just sprinkle what you've been given wherever you go. When you have love, you are filled, so there is plenty to go around. Sometimes others aren't as full as you and could use some more of what you have been freely given. ♡

Dear Lord, You have blessed me with so much love in my life. Loving parents, aunts, uncles, grandparents, cousins, friends, coworkers . . . the list goes on. I pray to spread this love and

share it with others because it has been freely given to me.
May more gentle, kind, and patient spirits walk this earth.
May they be the ones who rule! Oh, my God,
I LOVE YOU.

Be completely humble and gentle; be patient,
bearing with one another in love.

Ephesians 4:2 NIV

I FEED YOU

I recently heard someone say, "We are spiritual beings having a human experience," and I couldn't help but feel like an alarm went off in my mind. This statement truly spoke to me. Our life on earth 🌍 is so temporary. Our bodies will grow old and we will die, but our souls move on.

We are designed to have full, cheerful hearts. 🤍 The world may feel at times like it is overcome with nothing but pain, but God has made a way for us to live in His love no matter what happens to us on earth. 🌍

EVERY HUMAN deserves to have joy. If we fill our minds first with things we are grateful for and take time to acknowledge where all the blessings stem from, then we will be enlightened.

Our Creator feeds us with divine nutrients. If you eat His food and drink from His cup, you are strengthened spiritually, emotionally, and physically. With God, your well-being is no longer based on your circumstance, but rather how much space you allow for Him to fill. 🤍

Dear Father, I will continue to lose more people I love. My heart has more ache in store and my body will age, but none of this scares me anymore. You see, I have all I need. You are the wind under my wings, and because I have You, I have joy when I shouldn't. I have peace because it's You Who feeds me; please spread Your feast. I pray for lost souls to know Your table is open to all. Use me, I want to reach these souls, the ones who need

it the most. Thank You for feeding me; may I pass it along.
Help me answer Your call. I will take care of
Your sheep, and in doing this,
I FEED YOU.

His divine power has given us everything we need for
a godly life through our knowledge of him who called
us by his own glory and goodness.

2 Peter 1:3 NIV

I ENDURE FOREVER

I am working on bringing things to God in the moment so
I can gain His guidance as things are happening. Due to the nature
of His love—steadfast and enduring forever—I am able to move
forward **KNOWING** I am exactly where I am supposed to be and
not questioning the other five directions I could have gone.

God's love is steadfast, which means it is firm and
unwavering. When you make a decision based on
His love, you can **NEVER** go wrong. Our Creator is
so tender and is always there. His love is the greatest
comfort and is freely available to all.

Dear Father, Your steadfast love is what has gotten me through
the darkest of nights and coldest of days. My sweet Lord, as I grow
closer to You, I pray to learn more about Your nature. Make in me
an unwavering soul, who chooses light, love, and hope. Who
honors others and acts with compassion. Who loves with fire
and serves with a faithful heart. Lord, create in me a spirit,
one that dwells so close to You that
I ENDURE FOREVER.

For the LORD is good and his love endures forever; his
faithfulness continues through all generations.

Psalm 100:5 NIV

JULY

MY VIEW

Imagine if we could see all God sees. Imagine if we had a view from above, if we could sit on His cloud ☁ and watch people everywhere.

I'd see mothers with their morning coffee ☕, getting their children ready for school. People going for runs before work and enjoying happy hour with their friends after. Couples dining outside, eating a delicious meal. Parents rising with the sun, heading to work to feed their families.

On average, the majority of my time is spent at work. And after that, I have time to do whatever I want. I am slowly discovering what feeds me emotionally, spiritually, mentally, and physically.

What elevates your view? If you had a heavenly view of your life and could see it all from above, what are the things you would do more of? What do you do that elevates your mind? What do you do that makes your day worthwhile? We all have obligations, but with what little time you have to yourself, I encourage you to reflect on how you use it.

Knowing what makes you smile is important. It's so simple, it almost seems silly, but for most people who have obligations that extend beyond themselves, they probably do not know what makes them smile. And if they do, they don't spend enough time doing things that bring them true peace. ✨☕🤍

Dear God, You see it all. You see me wake with the sun, eat, sleep, walk, laugh, cry, and everything in between. My God, I pray for others to experience Your view from above. One that wakes their souls and warms their hearts. One that causes deep reflection and intention. My time on earth is oh so limited, please expand

MY VIEW.

For God watches how people live; He sees everything they do.

Job 34:21 NLT

EVERY INCH

I tend to compartmentalize my emotions. Create a box, draw a line, keep it clean, nice and organized . . . but that's not life, and that's not how God wants to move.

Sweet Vendy, allow Me to enter
every inch of your life
Allow My Spirit to enter every
conversation, interaction, and relationship
So there may be nothing but fullness
and love that surrounds your every move
My Spirit is all-powerful and untouchable

Invite in God's Spirit to fill every inch of your life and watch the transformation. Your reality, your heart, your mind, your body, **EVERYTHING.**

Dear Lord, it's hard for me to let go and trust. This morning I pray, please allow Your Spirit in. Please pour it out, Your supernatural presence. Spirit come 🤍 and take over my *EVERY INCH.*

Do you not know that you are God's temple
and that God's Spirit dwells in you?

1 Corinthians 3:16 ESV

WALK WITH ME

When we take time to walk with God, we see things in a different light. When I approach situations with an open mind and try my hardest to just listen, I end up taking away more than if I were talking.

When we walk with God, we become better at both listening and hearing. Our Creator knows every detail of our lives, and when we take time to rest and listen, we step into **MORE** truth, understanding, beauty, and wisdom than we could have ever found on our own.

When you walk with your Creator, He creates safe zones that cultivate rest so you can accomplish all He has placed on your heart. He brings truth and wisdom, so you are protected, **NOT** held back from all the desires He planted in your heart. He makes a path for your dreams.

Dear Lord, close my mouth and still my body so I can rest long enough to hear from You. You know my every move. When I wake, when I break, when I lie, when I cry, when I kiss, when I miss, when I dream, when I scream. God, I know if I make time for You, my life will be filled with more of Your fruit—more beauty, wisdom, and power. My God, You know the desires of my heart, so help me learn to walk with You. You Who has planned my life so masterfully, please always *WALK WITH ME.*

For we are His creation, created in Christ Jesus for good works, which
God prepared ahead of time so that we should walk in them.

Ephesians 2:10 HCSB

✦ *SIT IN MY BOAT* ✦

I protect the boat
I steer the boat
I decide who gets in the boat
And no matter what waters I lead you through
Rough or calm, deep or shallow, through strong winds
Hot days or cold days, rainy days, foggy days
Rivers or oceans
I am always in control of the boat

God's boat is the one you want to be in, and that's the beauty of life. No matter what the weather is or how rough the waters get, with the right perspective, through the lens of His truth, all the waters can be beautiful because you're sitting in the right boat—the one God is guiding.

You want to stay in the boat God has, for there you are protected. It's supernatural. It surpasses understanding.

For your heart ♡ to truly want to sit in that boat. For your heart to truly know. Sometimes you have to break. Sometimes your heart must break to choose to sit in His boat. The water has to overpower you. Then you will know, it was and always will be Him.

Life has to cut so deep that you are blessed with a realization that this fallen place is not worth riding the highs or lows, unless it's with the author of all that is good—the publisher of peace. When you sit in His boat, you will always be more than okay, no matter what water you journey through.

This world 🜨 is so temporary. Our hearts are created
for so much more. For all that's good. Dear broken
heart, please try and keep this in mind . . . we are all
just here for a very short time.

The good news is our souls will soon move on to that place, His
kingdom that is free of pain and suffering. But in the meantime,
choose to sit in God's boat. It is impossible to go wrong while
you are in your Creator's boat.

Dear Lord, I pray for more souls to experience what it is like to
sit in Your boat. For You to be the captain of their ship! I just know
once they experience Your truth, protections, wisdom, and might,
there will be no getting out of the boat. The vast sea is no match for
You! No matter what comes our way or shatters our hearts, I pray
we all choose to sit in Your boat. If that means I leave mine,
so be it. I no longer want to
SIT IN MY BOAT.

I know what it is to be in need, and I know what it is to have plenty. I have
learned the secret of being content in any and every situation, whether well
fed or hungry, whether living in plenty or in want. I can do all this
through Him who gives me strength.

Philippians 4:12-13 NIV

✶ LET GO ✶

Sometimes I feel the need to control situations that are close to my heart. When it comes to family, it's easy to forget that your family members are human too. They aren't perfect. And just because you are family, it doesn't always mean you're going to see eye to eye.

The older I get, the more independent I grow, and the more my worldview shifts and evolves. The more things and people change. It's easy to keep this in mind when I'm dealing with friends or people that aren't my family, but it's important to keep this in mind with family too.

It's okay to see things differently than the people you love the most. Love them and always want what's best for them, but know when to let go. Know you can't change the way someone views something if that hasn't been their experience or evolution.

Trust that God will take care, protect, and love that person in the place you can't seem to meet them. It's okay to let go in love. 🤍

Dear Father, I have such a hard time surrendering. Why do I crave control so much? Especially in such a broken world! Oh, Father, please help me let go. Speak to my heart and mind right now, show me the way to go, help me see, understand, or know so I can better
LET GO.

Do not let the sun go down while you are still angry.

Ephesians 4:26 NIV

ALL FROM ME

Reflecting this morning, I felt so grateful. Grateful for all the love I have in my life, all the support and the amazing humans I know. For my family, friends, and all the experiences I have had, the joy-filled memories I have.

As I continued to reflect on all I'm grateful for, the bad started to creep in. The bad is the pain of loss, hardships, or uncertainty, and hurt that comes with loving another human. I am learning what it means to be grateful for that too. For the pain I had to endure that was not my doing as well as for the pain I chose.

Our Creator is always in control, and though He does not inflict harm on His creation, He allows us to go through difficulties.

The hardships in my life have given me wisdom, strength, and **COMPASSION**.

We are more godlike when we endure pain.

The weight we once carried turns into wings. The struggles are what allow us to rise. With God, what was meant to end you only refines you.

We have the power to choose, even if it's as simple as how we choose to view our situations. And if you believe things randomly happen to you, know there is power in you choosing hope, faith, compassion, and love in any circumstance.

Dear Lord, You have blessed me with much. A loving
family I can always lean on, amazing friends that sweeten my life,
sunsets, coffee walks, and mighty dreams. I pray more souls learn
to embrace the hardships we walk through. I know some of my
sufferings were due to the decisions I made and others—I was a
sheep among wolves! Either way, I thank You today for my pain.
My pain allows me to fall deeply in love with You. The pain gave
me wings, grew my heart, and befriended wisdom. My God, I pray
others learn what it looks like to embrace their pain, leaving behind
the shame. Oh, my God, I now know after walking through the pain,
all that is good is from You. Father, since I now dwell so close to
You, I truly believe everything that happens to me is for a reason.
Reasons I do not always understand, but they allow me to soar on
wings like an eagle. So Lord, I ask that You use all of my
pain, may it be used for Your kingdom. Sprinkle it where
you wish, every ounce of it,
ALL FROM ME.

They will soar on wings like eagles.

Isaiah 40:31 NIV

NOTHING YOU DO

In the eyes of our Creator, we are like newborn babies. Like infants,
He holds us in His arms and supports our necks from flopping over.
We see the world, and there is so much we do not understand. As
infants we are powerless, and so much is out of our control.

I am sending you out like sheep among wolves.

Matthew 10:16 NIV

It's hard to imagine my 86-year-old grandfather as an infant, or
my 56-year-old mother and 27-year-old brother as just babies. The
wisest person you know, the person you look up to the most, is an
infant in the arms of God. He protects them in ways that are
unseen by the human eye.

There is nothing we can do that could stop God's
love for His innocent children, ones He created
and breathed to life. No matter what you do or say,
God sees you as innocent because there is so much
wisdom we lack, and our human bodies and
minds are **SO** limited.

All the good, everything you've been blessed with,
all the positive life moves, friends, family, the
beauty in your everyday life comes from a loving
Creator Who supports your neck the same way a
loving mother holds a newborn baby in her arms.

Dear Father, there is nothing we could have ever done to deserve this type of love, but it's a gift we are freely given. Help us seek more of Your love, wisdom, and words so our lives can be transformed as You open our eyes to Your power and glory. My God, help me remember it is all You, remove the worry, strip it from our minds for there is nothing to do.

Yes, sweet V,
NOTHING YOU DO.

Watch and pray so that you will not fall into temptation.
The spirit is willing, but the flesh is weak.

Matthew 26:41 NIV

INVITE ME IN

When worry overcomes me or I feel anxious about things
that are in the future, it hurts God. He doesn't like to see
His children worry. It robs us of our peace.

Usually when I start to worry, I begin to think of what I could
or should be doing so I can guarantee a certain result. And then
one thing happens that I did not expect, and there goes my
plan. Or it's an emotion that comes over me. It starts off small,
but one thought leads to another, and I've created this big story
based on fear of what could or might not happen.

To combat worry, I remove myself and go on a walk or take time
to talk to God. His presence takes away this worry, and I am able
to relax. He reminds me of what He has done and will continue to
do. He reminds me of His promises and what He stands for, which
then brings me peace. I can rest in His shade. His goodness is
just so rich.

Fear doesn't come from God. Worry doesn't come
from God. So emotions you feel that stem from
fear or worry do not produce logical answers. When
your emotions take over, invite God into your mind,
and focus on bringing your thoughts back to Him.

The Lord is not slow in keeping his promise, as some understand
slowness. Instead he is patient with you.

2 Peter 3:9 NIV

God is sovereign and gives according to His perfect
will for your life. It's **PERFECT**, which means
He is never late or slow. All we have to do is continue
to invite Him in. Invite Him in that very moment of
worry or doubt.

Dear Lord, I grow impatient, and as a result, I am robbed of my
peace. Please let me remember that You live in eternity, and my
finite human mind does not always understand Your time. Bring
comfort to my heart through Your love. I know, my God, the time
will pass, and You are never slow with Your promises but
rather oh so patient with me. Please continue to love me
through it, and always
INVITE ME IN.

Become complete. Be of good comfort, be of one mind, live in
peace; and the God of love and peace will be with you.

2 Corinthians 13:11 NKJV

BE YOU

When I asked my Creator what I can do for Him today,
His response was simple:
Be you.

I used to pull away from God's love because I felt pressure. I had
expectations of what it looked like to have a relationship with God,
and I was scared that my desires didn't match up with His. But the
truth is God just wants to love us, and for us to love Him. He
doesn't expect anything in return. And when you love, you naturally
want to please Him because you know how **GOOD** and true
He is. You know that He wants to bless you beyond belief.

When we are truly ourselves, it makes God
happy. He created us in His image, and we
are made perfect because of all He has done.

What does being yourself look like?

You are strong and confident. You are able to love on people because
you know how loved you are. He causes your cup to bubble over.
You carry a lightness because you know the Creator—the most
powerful being—is on your side and working to weave together the
most beautiful life for you, regardless of your circumstance. Give
yourself permission to walk with joy and be full today, for He, my
dear, has already made the way!

Walk without fear and in courage.

Dear God, thank You for all You have done. Today I can walk in courage, fearless, because I know Your perfect love casts away my fears. By and through You, fear is no longer welcomed. It no longer has power over me, and this, my sweet Lord, brings You mighty joy. I pray for others to experience this freedom, freedom to be godlike, freedom to experience You in their daily lives. Our mighty Savior You are. You create in us something new, something that reflects You. I pray to live a life that has more of You. A life where I become one with Your Spirit, to

BE YOU.

For the LORD your God is living among you. He is a mighty savior.
He will take delight in you with gladness. With his love,
he will calm all your fears.

Zephaniah 3:17 NLT

✦ *I'M EXCITED* ✦

My favorite prayer is the "Our Father." It's short and precise.
It covers all the bases and it is pure truth.

Our Father which art in heaven, Hallowed be thy name. Thy kingdom come, Thy will
be done on earth, as it is in heaven. Give us this day our daily bread. And forgive us our
debts, as we forgive our debtors. And lead us not into temptation, but deliver us from evil:
For thine is the kingdom, and the power, and the glory, for ever. Amen.

Matthew 6:9-13 KJV

Until now I never gave "Your kingdom come, your will be done, on
earth as it is in heaven" much thought. It's always my prayer over
my own life for God's will to be done because I know He has best,
but His will to be done on earth, all over? In this place where there is
so much suffering for so many people? **HOW?** I can accept that our
souls are made for more and that we will one day be in the heavenly
realm with our Creator, but a world 🌍 where there is more
light than darkness?

God is excited. He is moving in the hearts of His people,
and it's powerful. His way, His light, is getting ready to
take over in unprecedented ways.

His true, **GOOD** will is coming and will be done. I know when God
moves in my life, it's powerful, and I can't close my eyes or ignore
His love because it's the only thing that gets me through.Our Creator
is on the move, and He is getting ready to pour out His Spirit.
His light is going to touch lives all over.

So get ready! And ask God to guide you in your hopes
and dreams that are in line with His will. 🤍

Dear God, Prince of Peace and Mighty Shepherd for all who seek. I pray to You this morning, asking that Your will be done in my life and those who bend a knee to You! My God, I want to see You flip the script. I want to see a mighty move by, in, and through Your Spirit for all Your people. Please Father, thy kingdom come, thy will be done on earth as it is in heaven. Eek,

I'M EXCITED!

For I will pour water on the thirsty land, and streams on the dry ground;
I will pour out my Spirit on your offspring, and my blessing
on your descendants.

Isaiah 44:3 NIV

FOCUS ON ME

When we focus on God, we worry less about what will happen to us because we know He is in control and does it all. When we focus on our Creator and His plan, there is less striving and rushing to check things off our list to the point where we miss life. When we focus on God, we get to experience more doors opening naturally. We can experience a deep sense of peace, which allows us to move forward through the right door, not only with a willingness, but with a gracious and humble spirit because we know it **WASN'T** our doing. As a result, this humble spirit causes you to flourish where He places you.

This is challenging for me to wrap my mind around because I enjoy the striving at times. But the striving causes me to burn out more quickly and push important relationships to the side because I am not able to water them the way I would like to.

God is love and His core is all that is good, all that is good that has happened to you. He just wants to see His people live full, blessed, abundant lives. We get there by focusing on Him and less on our surroundings. Less on our purpose and more on supporting people whose hearts are in the right place.

Work hard at all you do, and He can use it all for His glory, but be humble and gracious enough to know it's not really your doing, but your loving Creator's doing. He will do all the major stuff, you just gotta keep your thoughts focused on His love and goodness and, most importantly, be willing. That way you are full and pour from a full cup, not an empty one.

Dear God, I desire Your will so strongly; however, I know
I cannot accomplish Your will on my own. The water You call me to
walk through, the mountains You'd like me to climb, the vision You
give me—I must hold Your hand, and You must lead the way. I know
You will equip me to accomplish all You set before me, but only if
I focus on You. Please fill my mind with Your thoughts and remove
mine. Mine are of the flesh, they are limited by what they see and
know, but Your thoughts, Your ways are all higher than mine.
Help me focus on You and not
FOCUS ON ME.

Stop striving and know that I am God; I will be exalted among
the nations, I will be exalted on the earth.

Psalm 46:10 NASB

✴ *TAKE ME WITH YOU* ✴

Everywhere you go, you have access to God's Spirit; He has the
power to live in you. No matter where you go, whether it be
church or a night out with your friends, you can invite
His Spirit to come with you.

I like to invite God's Spirit in the mornings because I feel safe after.
I feel protected when His Spirit is with me. I feel like I'm less likely
to do something silly that I may regret later, or speak and act in a
way that doesn't reflect His truth and light.

No matter what you're doing, or where you're going,
ask God's Spirit to join you. To guide you, even if it's
just through the day. You will be able to go to bed and
have peace, knowing every human interaction was
handled with love and grace, with the fruits of His Spirit.

When you take your Creator's Spirit with you each day
as you step out the door, you'll stop running over
interactions in your head and smile, knowing
He was with you the entire time. 🖤

Dear Lord, there is no place I want to venture without You. Please
send your Spirit to guide me today. Send Your Spirit with me so
I may walk with a light that is seen by others. Send Your Spirit
with me so I can bring healing to those I meet through kindness.
Transform me with Your gentle Spirit, give me wisdom that
fills a room, please please please
TAKE ME WITH YOU.

Yet I am always with you; you hold me by my right hand.

Psalm 73:23 NIV

PROXIMITY TO ME

Proximity = nearness or closeness.

This morning I wanted to know when I'll be ready for all
the beautiful things that have been put on my heart. 🩶 I wanted
God to give me a timeline. My Creator said,
It's based on your proximity to Me.

When you are close to Me
When you spend time with Me and
hold My hand for every step
Allowing My Spirit to guide you to the point where
You trust Me more than you doubt
When you surrender what you want most and have peace
Then you will be ready, sweet V

So, the timeline of all I dream really depends on me?

It's not a matter of "if" but "when." The "if" God has full
control over. The "when" is all on us.

The timeline for all that God has for you does not depend
on the qualifications this world sets. The Creator of this
world has power over all things. Things like age,
experience, or time do not apply to you. The only thing
that does is your Creator's nearness to you.

Don't let anyone look down on you because you are young, but
set an example for the believers in speech, in conduct, in love,
in faith and in purity.

1 Timothy 4:12 NIV

Your proximity to your Creator determines your strength: strength to keep going when you want to stop, strength to take risks, and strength to stay put when you want to leave. The relationship you build with God strengthens your sense of direction, which becomes second nature due to the sensitivity to God's Spirit heightened in you.

Draw close and give God more time in whatever ways you **ENJOY**! Going for a walk, reading, or watching things that inspire you to grow closer to Him, creating a quiet space in the mornings, at night before bed, or in the bubble bath. Whatever it may look like for you, don't be afraid to pour into that time and **ASK** God whatever you want!

Dear God, the closer I grow to You, the more I realize how much time I need with You. The less I crave things of this world and the more I crave You. I pray others learn to give You more of their time so they will not only be strengthened but highly enlightened. Father, the timeline of all You have for me and all that is good, is surely due to my proximity to You. Please help me choose You each and every day. I don't want to miss out on a single thing You have for me. You are too good and so good to me. Please forever keep a close
PROXIMITY TO ME.

Study this Book of Instruction continually. Meditate on it day and night so you will be sure to obey everything written in it. Only then will you prosper and succeed in all you do.

Joshua 1:8 NLT

✦ *I BATHE YOU* ✦

I love a clean room and sitting in the bubble bath. When my room is clean, I feel mentally organized. I also love to take bubble baths. When I'm stressed, sad, or just want to relax, I take a bubble bath and I always feel better after.

Both these things are mental for me. Just because I have a clean room doesn't mean I'm productive, but I feel that way. And just because I take a bath doesn't mean my problems go away, but I feel restored.

When I bathe, I sit in the bubble bath for pleasure—not because I feel dirty and want to wash off. I enjoy sitting, relaxing and always feel rejuvenated after. That's what our Creator does to us. He bathes us to make us feel better. When God bathes you, He washes you. His water is so pure, it restores you.

You are best fully naked . . . vulnerable with God. Do not rush Him as He bathes you. He created you and knows everything, so your naked body (vulnerabilities) is a beautiful sight to Him.

He created our hearts like the sun and the earth. To stay in orbit, the sun ☀ must be at the center. It's a wise investment to seek God daily, not for His pleasure but for our own. I sometimes don't take a bath because of time or excuses I make, but I'm realizing the more I make time for simple things that restore me, the better I am when I go out into the world. The same is true with God. The more you make time to soak up His loving presence, the better you orbit.

Dear God, You bathe me daily, and as a result, my vulnerabilities have been transformed and my wounds are bandaged. You have restored me in a way that makes me crave You. Your presence is what I need to orbit. Thank You for giving me rest and making me feel better when I am sad, lonely, or hurting. May I learn to bathe You in my daily. I pray for others to bathe with You. Use me, whatever You need, may *I BATHE YOU*.

Come, let us return to the LORD. He has torn us to pieces; now he will heal us. He has injured us; now he will bandage our wounds. In just a short time he will restore us, so that we may live in his presence.

Hosea 6:1-2 NLT

I WEAVE TOGETHER

God wants to create a beautiful life for us filled with blessings beyond belief. Sometimes we are our own worst enemies and get in our own way.

How do we avoid this?

Live in the present moment. Slow down, take a moment or two in your day to reflect and say thank you. Reflect and feel. Reflect and see. Reflect and taste. He is taking care of it, and He just wants us to be present, to be still enough to know He is working and moving so you don't have to.

Practice being mindful and seeing all the good, the small things and the big things, because one thing we can **NEVER** get back in life is time. It comes and it goes.

Soak up the good in each day and more will come. When you are mindful and aware, the practice itself allows you to recognize everyday blessings in a more powerful way.

Dear God, my Master Weaver, You have never failed me. I have failed You many times, and yet You continue to restore me. I don't fully understand Your love, but I never question its goodness. How could I? You have been too good to me. Even in my most broken state, You continued to make a way, one that caused me to look up and to You. In dry wastelands, You continue to meet me, a pathway through the wilderness, You have always made. Thank You for all You have done, all You continue to do, and all You will

do. I thank You in advance for what's already mine. Help me be still long enough to join You, and by Your side, I will help You bring it all together, the beautiful plans from above for humans everywhere! Father, pick me. I want to join Your team, I want to help. Enlist me, choose me, train me! I will join You and I will help bring to motion mighty plans because You make me like You! So like You,
I WEAVE TOGETHER.

But forget all that—it is nothing compared to what I am going to do. For I am about to do something new. See, I have already begun! Do you not see it? I will make a pathway through the wilderness. I will create rivers in the dry wasteland.

Isaiah 43:18-19 NLT

✷ *RAIN DOWN* ✷

I was very fortunate growing up, surrounded by so much love from my family. I come from a big Mexican and Italian family, so family dinners with delicious food and quality time truly shaped me as a little girl. I remember my Nunu telling me, "To whom much is given, much is expected," and it would excite me! I have always wanted to make an impact in this world, create change, help others in some way, but now I hear this and it scares me.

When you live a blessed life with food, shelter, love, safety, and opportunity, you are meant to share it. Whatever influence you have in the world 🌎 , whatever ways you have been blessed, you are not to hold on so tightly to those gifts out of fear that they may not always be there. Rather, you expand on your blessing by blessing someone who is in more need than you. You share the knowledge, love, money, opportunity, support, or whatever it is you have been freely given. Not only does it come back to you more bountiful than before, but you are no longer enslaved or live with the fear of not having.

God entrusts people who give with **MORE**.

If you have been blessed and taken care of all your life, stop and think where that came from. None of us can control the the families we were born into or the cards we have been dealt from birth. We view our lives through a certain lens, and that perspective shapes how we act.

What have you been freely given? In return, what do you give?

I have found the more I give freely from the heart,
the more good comes my way.

As your blessings grow in life, you will have more
responsibility. All that is good and true in your life
comes from a higher power that has protected you in
ways you do not see. When you live with this
understanding and are guided by this truth, you give
freely because you know you have been blessed, and
God wants nothing more than for you to be a blessing
to someone else the same way He has blessed you.
He will continue to rain down on your life and
those around you in profound ways.

Dear God, oh the many ways You have blessed me. Keep my eyes
focused on this, especially on the days I fail to see all I have and all
You have done. I know, Lord, You will require much of me because
of how You have opened my eyes. My God, I know the measure
I use on others is not always fair, so please have mercy on me and
continue to grow me to do and be better. Through and because of
Your love, I will be a blessing to others. Healing will flow
because You have given me power to
RAIN DOWN.

Give to others, and God will give to you. Indeed, you will receive a full measure,
a generous helping, poured into your hands—all that you can hold. The measure
you use for others is the one that God will use for you.

Luke 6:38 GNT

FOCUS ON LOVE

I tend to get complacent, which leads to wanting more. I then start striving for things I don't need or get distracted from the path God has put me on.

How do I combat this?

Love. Focus on love, taking care of the people, the job, the things God has put in your life at whatever stage you are in. Then, in His time, you will eventually reach a point where He says, "Okay, time to move on to what I have next for you."

It's important to take care of what's on your plate now, in the current season you are in, because if you're not careful, you'll start adding things that He hasn't called you to add, which may hurt the blessing you already have or the one He is preparing for you.

When love and gratitude are at the center of all you do, your motives will be pure and you will be on the right track. I promise God will do the rest; He will send the people that are supposed to be in your life at the right time, and He will direct your next step.

How do we spot the "right time"?

He will give you peace. And you'll know it's the right time when you don't want whatever it is so much that you're holding it too tight or above Him. The right time is key because it ensures you have enough grace to keep what is to come next. Dear God, there

are things I have chased with You and things I have chased without You. I have experienced both to know, wish for, and pray every single day that it is Your will, Your time, Your reason, and Your rhyme I want more than anything. There have been times where I wanted the blessings more than You, and I am so sorry for the way that has hurt You. But, my God, I am learning the stronger I grow in Your love, the less my flesh seeks these blessings above You. I know, all I need is to
FOCUS ON LOVE.

And it is my prayer that your love may abound more and more, with knowledge and all discernment.

Philippians 1:9 ESV

✦ *I FILL YOU* ✦

Have you ever been around someone who walks into a room, and you can feel their energy? Or maybe just being around that person causes you to worry less?

I believe people like this, people with joy-filled souls, realize and truly understand that only God has the power to turn everything that happens to you in life into a blessing.

Relying on your own thinking and planning just makes you more anxious. Our true security lies with our Creator, the all-powerful God Who knows every detail of our future and what will happen before it even happens! When we look to Him, wait on Him, and ask for His guidance, we are filled.

Dear Lord, create in me a joy-filled soul. One that lifts others up, one that is used to advance Your kingdom and will on earth. Father, I love it when You hold my hand and guide me through; flowing from You is the wisest counsel a girl could have! You are my strength and my portion forever. I pray for more souls—lonely, broken, empty, and grief-filled souls—to choose You so they can be filled. I want to fill like You. Do something new in me, make it so I always choose You. Please, may
I FILL YOU.

Yet I am always with you; you hold me by my right hand. You guide me with your counsel, and afterward you will take me into glory. Whom have I in heaven but you? And earth has nothing I desire besides you. My flesh and my heart may fail, but God is the strength of my heart and my portion forever.

Psalm 73:23-26 NIV

✦ FACE TO FACE ✦

My sweet Vendy, I want
My children to know that I'm always here
I want them to know that I care,
that any questions they have, I'm here
That I do not change, My nature is consistent and the only
thing they can truly rely on
That I protect them always and they often don't see it
That I love them and the soft whisper is Me
And unlike humans,
My love never runs out, I am eternal

Our Creator is always there, and because of Jesus, we can have intimacy with Him—with the greatest power there is. Quiet yourself. Give it time and you will see.

Dear God, create in me a faith that believes in what I do not see. I know with You the reward for this kind of faith, faith in the unseen, is to then see what we believe. My dear God, pour down Your Spirit, send down Your warrior angels, let us see! For there is too much injustice, pain, and greed. Too much and at times this world feels too heavy for me. I want to see good win in this world and evil flee! I want more of your children—sweet little boys and girls, teens, all the mothers- and fathers-to-be—to experience You. I pray for more *FACE TO FACE.*

Every good gift, every perfect gift, comes from above. These gifts come
down from the Father, the creator of the heavenly lights, in whose character
there is no change at all.

James 1:17 CEB

I CONSUME YOU

Consume = to ingest,
take into the body by swallowing or absorbing.

If we are on a plate, we should want God to be the only
thing we allow to consume us.

What does that look like?

You living a full life filled with love for people, family, friends,
passion for work, zest for walking in your purpose and calling
because the Creator is the only thing you allow to consume You.

I struggle with keeping God first in my life and heart.
God, how do I allow You to consume me?

Put God first in all the ways you love with family,
friends, and people. He will make sure there is
enough to go around.

Every little thing that worries you, every little thing
that confuses you, bring to Him **FIRST**.

Wait on your Creator. His timing is never off, so be
patient and hopeful in faith. Speak whatever you are
hoping for Him to do with words that are filled with
truth and love.

Dear Lord, I pray to ingest more of You. My God, I get so
consumed so easily with things that do not feed me. Thoughts that
take over and are not from You. Please show us how to place you

first. Show us how to love like You, how to consult You first with the matters that weigh heavy on our hearts. Help us wait on You, God. Your timing is divine and manifests things in my life I could have never seen. Your timing points to the heavens. Your timing opens people's eyes. Oh, my God, please take over. Steer my ship. I invite Your Spirit in, Your guidance, and the beauty of wisdom. Oh, how it enables me to walk with grace and honor. My plate and everything I have on it is for You; may

I CONSUME YOU.

Seek the LORD and his strength; seek his presence continually!

1 Chronicles 16:11 ESV

✦ *CELEBRATE YOUR LIFE* ✦

God is leading me into a new chapter. After experiencing my loss, I'm starting to turn a corner—one with less grieving and more life.

Sometimes when we go through extremely painful things, we want to hide from the world; it's almost like shame is part of the pain. The crazy thing is that God wants us to be confident in our suffering. To know that we are growing in compassion and our eyes are being opened as He renews our souls. Prior to losing my dad, that was never my outlook on pain.

Our Creator uses every ounce of your pain for **GOOD**. God wants us to celebrate our lives, especially after we have weathered a storm.

First, forgive yourself and others. Forgive yourself for every little thing so you can be free, and forgive others so you won't be chained by living in offense. Forgiveness is for you, designed to free you.

Do more of, and make more time for, the things that make you smile. There is no need to ever make yourself small for other people; one way to break away from this is by doing more of what makes you smile. Why? Not only do you inspire others, but you're a better version of yourself and you give more to the world by doing simple things that bring you peace. With God, oftentimes He turns those simple things that bring you joy into big things . . .

God will take all you've been through and transform you; your soul will be a bright burning light in the world if you hand over your pain to Him. A light that gives off hope to others, but also a light that lives with depth because you have perspective and know both the good and bad that takes place under His sun. So never be ashamed of your pain, and when you can, share it with others; you will bring so much comfort to their hearts.

Your Creator wants to bring you through the hard stuff so you can have a much more full life. He wakes us up so we can smell, taste, see, and hear. And He wants us to **CELEBRATE** the good and the bad because of all He can do with it.

Dear Lord, there have been times in my life where I should have allowed more of the weeping and did not. There have been times when I should have laughed but held back. Times where I should have mourned but ran. Times where I wanted to dance and didn't. My God, I am making my way out of the most challenging season of my life, weathering the loss of my dad. You have shown me that the dark will come just like the light, and when it's all said and done, all will be okay because it is You Who makes the way, brings healing, holds us, and brings blessings beyond belief. My Lord, there is a time and a season for everything under Your sun, so teach me, show me what it looks like to celebrate. Teach me how to have joy again. You made a way when there was no way, and now it's time for me to lift up my praise. I want to celebrate the life You have given me. I want to *CELEBRATE YOUR LIFE.*

A time to weep, and a time to laugh; a time
to mourn, and a time to dance.

Ecclesiastes 3:4 ESV

DESIGNED FOR MORE

Humans have souls and our souls are what go on. We are designed for more than just our experience and time on earth. 🌐 We are designed for more.

More than the pain, more than the joy, we are created in our Creator's image. He is eternal; therefore, we have a seed planted in our hearts for things that are eternal. Love is one of those things. There will never be a "right time" to lose someone you love. And our desire to live in peace, a place that is absent from suffering, is a desire every human has. Yet, it makes no sense because that will never happen on earth—nor has it ever happened—because we all hurt each other. I believe we crave this because our eternal Father has created this place called heaven. Heaven, unlike our fallen world, is free from suffering and is a destination for our souls.

So while we are here, the way we treat others is really the only thing that matters. The act of kindness left undone is what you will regret because the act of kindness is what touches one's soul. It's what brings healing. Our Lord, the Mighty Creator of all, delights in kindness.

Dear Lord, don't let the sun set leaving so much undone. I pray for more tender words, more letters of gratitude and appreciation, and more flowers sent. My God, it's not the things we do but the things left undone that birth heartache. So please teach me, teach others, how we are so greatly *DESIGNED FOR MORE.*

"...And if anyone gives even a cup of cold water to one of these little ones who is my disciple, truly I tell you, that person will certainly not lose their reward."

Matthew 10:42 NIV

NO ONE LIKE ME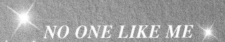

There is no one like God. There is no one life that is the same. We all have a unique formula to our creation. We have a different set of life experiences that make up our worldview, a different set of parents, a uniquely shaped heart, a variety of emotions. Every human is unique.

There is no one who is able to love you like your Creator. He gives you rest and protects you in many ways you can't see. He knows exactly what you need to hear and what you don't. He knows the true desires of your heart and your every fear.

Ask God to give you His formula because no human has the power, ability, or knowledge to give you what you need like the Creator of all.

Each and every moment of every day, He knows exactly what you need—more than you even know. What better choice do we have than to choose our Creator's love? It is something we can't get anywhere else; it's divine and all-powerful.

All you have to do is ask and you will receive.

Dear God, I do not fully understand the way You have created me. I feel set apart at times, my heart hurts because I do not always like what I see. I feel that the ways of this world are not always for me. But then You come, You show me what I need to see, speak to me, and help me understand all I truly need is You. You to see, You to thrive, You to live, grow, and be. Please, God, continue to create in me a unique soul, a person who dwells so close to You, it is recognized in this world that is far from You. Oh, God, I know we are all different, we have different strengths, different weaknesses, but I thank You for all that makes us different because it points back to You. You hold the keys; You have the perfect formula to feed. I love how You have created

NO ONE LIKE ME.

Ask and it will be given to you; seek and you will find; knock and the door will be opened to you. For everyone who asks receives; the one who seeks finds; and to the one who knocks, the door will be opened.

Matthew 7:7-8 NIV

AUGUST

✦ I AM YOUR AUTHOR ✦

I find much comfort and joy in knowing that there is a greater power weaving together a plan for my life, resulting in the greatest glory and good.

The hard part is believing this in the midst of confusion, hurt, pain, and the unknown. It's only rational to want to take matters into our own hands when we experience hardship, but that's not what we are called to do.

Let your Creator fight every battle for you. Our only job is to focus on His love, truth, and light. God will do the rest. Our Creator produces justice for His people; He just asks that we stand back and truly trust Him in the middle of it all. He will go before your every step.

Dear Lord, You have told me of the many promises You have for me. Many I have yet to see. Some days it is easier for me to believe and trust than others. On the days I lack trust and faith in You, I feel I must do more, which usually just ends up exhausting me or placing me outside Your will—and I never want anything that is not Your will for me. You, my God, are the greatest author for me. May I always choose You, pick up Your pen, and trust the way You write. I know with You each chapter is new, different, and usually better than the last! Thank You, God. I love You, and I pray to hand these next steps over to You. May Your will and only Your will be done. Please just take me by the hand, show me how to pick up the pen, and together let's write so the world can see a mighty move—a mighty outpouring of Your Spirit.

I, Vendela Raquel, will write for You; I work for You;
I AM YOUR AUTHOR.

I am with you and will watch over you wherever you go, and I will
bring you back to this land. I will not leave you until I have done
what I have promised you.

Genesis 28:15 NIV

I AM GOD

I created all things
I am all-powerful
I know no limits
I see all things
I defeated death
I make new
I am the One and Only

God lives in each of us and with this powerful source in us, nothing is impossible. Yet I tend to look at situations in my life and put them in a box so I can feel like I understand them. This creates limits and boundaries on what I can do because I am leaving out the worldview of my Creator.

A living and powerful God wants to see you transform and be renewed by His hand. Invite your Creator in so you can **SEE** all the possibilities.

With God, there is less conforming and more becoming.

With God, life has more color and greater meaning. God wants us to be excited and hopeful for all the wonderful things to come. He also wants us to be grateful and love where we are at. If we only understood how great and limitless God is, we would all live differently.

Dear Lord, there is nothing You have not done for me. There is much I have not done for You, and because of this, I am sure I have missed out on certain blessings You have designed for me.

That is the horrible part of choice and free will. Because I get to choose You each and every day, there are many opportunities to not choose You. And when I don't choose You, I choose a life that falls short of Your mighty will. Your good, true, beautiful, and amazing will! My God, Your thoughts are higher than my thoughts, and Your ways are higher than my ways. I know in my heart that I want You and Your will, so please help me choose You. My Lord, I am excited for who I am becoming as I grow closer to You and learn what it looks like to choose You each day. You are my God, and the closer we grow, the more near You dwell, for You are the God in me; divine You make me. Thank You for the power that is at work in me because of He Who came and He, Your Son, Who said,

I AM GOD.

Now to him who is able to do immeasurably more than all we ask or imagine, according to his power that is at work within us.

Ephesians 3:20 NIV

ENJOY TODAY

God's grace is more than enough to get us through whatever we face, especially if we take it day by day. I often look down at my phone, and I can't believe how fast the months have flown by. Life moves so quickly and there is no stopping time, ever.

Enjoy the car ride or walk to pick up your morning coffee, the breeze that sweeps, and the afternoon spent with someone you care for. Enjoy the sun hitting your face, getting ready for the day, playing your favorite song on repeat, creating a delicious meal, and eating a delicious meal. Enjoy the people and love you have in your life because today will never come again.

Seasons will come when you are blessed with more. As a result, you will look back and crave the simple things you used to have more time to enjoy.

Our lives on earth 🌎 are so short and go by so fast. There will always be a time when you wish you could have enjoyed a moment, person, or experience more. Now is the only and best time. Just enjoy today.

The practice of enjoying each day results in a lifetime full of memories and gratitude that bubbles over and makes your heart warm, especially on the days you need those memories most. 🤍

Dear Lord, I know You desire for me to have joy each day. I know it hurts You when I worry or move through life as if today will come again. I know You wish to open my eyes every day to the joy that lies in the simple things. I know that as the seasons of life change and You fill my life with more blessings, I will be tempted to lose sight of You. My season of healing has taught me many things, but one thing I desire to always ring true is finding joy in the simple things of each day. My morning cup of matcha, a fresh meal, or a sunset walk. My God, I pray more hearts and minds become open to daily rituals that will transform how they go through life.

My God, I pray to simply

ENJOY TODAY.

I know that there is nothing better for people than to be happy and to do good while they live. That each of them may eat and drink, and find satisfaction in all their toil—this is the gift of God.

Ecclesiastes 3:12-13 NIV

PRAISE ME

Praise is vital when preparing for, or expecting, something
special to happen in your life.

God doesn't need our praise but when we praise Him, we are
showing trust in His power, releasing our fear and anxiety in the
present moment and creating space for Him to move. We are
creating a zone for Him to better work and open the door. We are
creating space for Him to perform the miracle.

Our spiritual power is in proportion to our faith. The more we
feed our faith, the stronger we become and the more of
God's Spirit can live in each of us. Praise feeds our faith.

Whatever you are preparing for—an interview, special date, or
any event—try thanking God in advance for what you are
about to receive. He moved in the past, and He will do it again. And
again. And again. Because your Creator knows no limits and lives
beyond anything you could ever imagine or think of for yourself.

Dear God, I thank You in advance for what I am about to receive.
I thank You for all You have done and continue to do. I pray I am
able to lay it down as easily as I received it. I pray to take good care
of the people and experiences You are going to bless me with, and
I thank You for teaching me the power in Your praise. Because of
the way You have moved in and covered me, I receive glory
I do not deserve, but I thank You for the ways You
PRAISE ME.

Heal me, LORD, and I will be healed; save me and
I will be saved, for you are the one I praise.

Jeremiah 17:14 NIV

SPIN YOUR WORLD

The world is constantly spinning. We live in a place where, if we are not intentional and do not force ourselves to slow down and smell, taste, see, love, and feel, it will all pass by.

Let God control your tempo so that, as the world continues to spin, you will be better equipped to hold on to the important things. When God decides to pick up the speed, the only way for you to keep up is by living close to Him.

Choose your Creator because nothing compares to the life He can create for you. God will show you that no amount of pain or suffering will compare to all He has in store for you. The beauty, joy, and pure bliss that comes from Him makes all that you have gone through small. Even your sufferings become small—this is something only God has the power to do.

Dear Lord, I know You have the power to hold this world in the palm of Your hand. I find that on the days I do not sit with You, my world starts to spin out of control. I move through my day rushing, and anxiety starts to creep in. My God, I know there is nothing You cannot do because I personally have experienced You move on my behalf time and time again, and yet my faith is small. God, I pray for the souls who need to read this today. I lift up those souls to You who go through life and miss it all. They miss the mark and labor with a burning heat to their back because they feel the work of their hands is all on them. The pressure of the spinning world weighs extra heavy on the souls that live far from You. Lord, I pray You continue to create pure hearts to walk this earth blamelessly,

lacing each step with sweet victory that points to Your justice and beauty. My God, take over new grounds, take over new spaces, places, and spheres as You continue to
SPIN YOUR WORLD.

He will make your innocence radiate like the dawn, and the justice of your cause will shine like the noonday sun.

Psalm 37:6 NLT

I KNOW EVERY DESIRE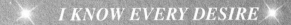

We all have a unique set of gifts and talents. Sometimes it takes a severe blow to awaken our gifts, a trial that pushes us forward so we can grow in ways we would have never grown otherwise.

The more life I live, the truer I find this to be. We all have desires that have been placed on our hearts ♡ since we were young. Depending on what stage we are currently in, some of us know exactly what they are, some of us have no idea, and some of us are in the middle.

If you see your life through God's lens, you will be hopeful, courageous, and faithful as you navigate the desires of your heart. He will give you this lens because that's His promise: to give life and life abundantly.

Most of us have dreams. Sometimes we don't even know what they are, but we can feel something there pushing us, making us reach higher when we don't want to. This is usually God's calling in your life. Protect it by seeking a relationship with your Creator because sometimes even people you love will not be able to see it. Not because they don't believe in you, but because it's between you and your Creator.

Dear Lord, planted in me is a deep desire, a desire for You, a desire for justice, love, peace, and an unraveling of much I cannot see. I have always felt Your call in my life, but I have not always followed it. My God, You took my dad from me at the age of twenty-three because You knew it would force me to my knees. You knew it would grow my heart for You. You knew it would awaken gifts in me all from You. You knew it would train and prepare me for the desires planted in me. God, thank You for the training that takes place in each of us by Your hand. You sent Your Son many years ago to earth. When He left, He took with Him the keys of Hades; He defeated death so we could claim the victory. Yes, it's true, He wears them around His neck! My God, I now have life and life abundantly.

I now walk in more freedom, and I have risen from the ashes of death that brought pain so heavy it once covered my innocent heart in shame. My God, I pray for your people everywhere, may You use their pain, free them from the shame, and speak to the depths of their hearts as they search for healing. May You, my God, do for them what You did for me in the midst of my deepest grief. Speak to the desires of their hearts. Show them the beautiful plans You have for them so they can keep going. Tell them of the victory that was won over two thousand years ago by Your Son so their faint hearts can keep a steady pace in the race. May they not fall behind due to their pain, but do what You did for me: use it to empower them! It's You Who brought comfort to my heart when no human could, it's You Who told me to keep going and said,

Sweet Vendy, I have the keys.
I KNOW EVERY DESIRE.

I came that they may have life and have it abundantly.

John 10:10 ESV

MORE THAN ENOUGH

You are more than enough for God to love you. You are more than enough to accomplish anything you want. Everyone is chosen, but not everyone chooses.

When you choose, you are transformed. Here's the catch: It's a choice we must make every day for the rest of our lives.

Choosing God is something we must do daily. You are worthy to choose His love and receive all that comes along with that choice. It may feel hard at first but the more times you choose His love, the stronger you grow and the more you are willing to choose Him again and again.

With God, you are never alone and you don't have to do anything alone. He is always there to support and guide you. You just have to ask and choose Him.

Dear God, Your Spirit has made me more patient, tender, and pure. I see things differently—with more compassion and clarity. I am stronger yet more meek. I believe I am more than enough because of Your sweet, consistent love that rains over me. I pray more of Your creation experiences this by choosing You daily and learning what it looks like to sit and wait on You. My God, You make us *MORE THAN ENOUGH.*

For he chose us in him before the creation of the world
to be holy and blameless in his sight. In love.

Ephesians 1:4 NIV

I AM GATEKEEPER

With your Creator, nothing happens by chance. When you dwell close to God, He protects you in mystical ways. When you walk by His side, He becomes your gatekeeper. That means nothing randomly happens to you. Every human you meet, every face you recognize, every name you recall—there is a reason for it.

When God is the gatekeeper for your life, no one gets in without His permission. Every human interaction, He has planned. He knows exactly how you will feel, and since His ways are higher than ours, this is the ultimate protection.

Every door closed is a blessing in the **EXACT** same way every open door is a blessing. They are all part of a much greater plan.

There is more opportunity to feed certain relationships and less opportunity for others. When you truly hand it over to Him, every step of your life is part of a divine plan much greater than you. A plan so great you could have **NEVER** dreamed of it yourself, let alone made it happen.

Hand your key over to the greatest gatekeeper there is. Your Creator will transform you—your life, soul, mind, and body—into a reflection of His love and power. There is nothing you cannot do with God.

Dear God, I pray today for more of the impossible to be possible by Your hand. Take the key to my heart, mind, and spirit. You are now my gatekeeper, and because of this my path is lit. I pray to be Yours, and since I belong to You, I will look after Your sheep. Help me, show me, Lord, how to take good care of Your sheep. Lace my steps with hope, love, and faith. Appoint me to new levels—mighty levels. With You, Lord,

I AM GATEKEEPER.

Jesus replied, "The things that are impossible for people are possible for God."

Luke 18:27 ISV

MY BLESSINGS

Whatever is in front of you today, enjoy it. A loving mother, an iced latte, a sunny day, a rest-filled weekend, your favorite show, a wonderful friend, a loving family—whatever it may be.

Enjoy it because it's yours to enjoy and tomorrow it may not be there. Don't ever feel bad for your blessings, enjoy them! Take a moment to take them in and say thank You. It could all be gone tomorrow, but the experience, the love and joy it brought you, will live forever and continue to shape your heart. 🤍
The impact will last.

Much has changed in my life over such a short period of time, and I can now see how powerful and good our Creator truly is. He doesn't always give you what you want, but He will always give you more than enough of what you need.

Today God wants me to know it's okay to enjoy all I have been blessed with—both past and current blessings. He wants us to know that different seasons call for different blessings. What is there one day may not be there the next, but that's not the point. The point is to enjoy it while you have it and know that God will always take care of you, no matter where you are at in life.

Dear Lord, I have asked much of You and from You. I do not always understand Your timeline, or why You allow certain things to take place in this world, but I do trust You to always provide for me. There is not one thought of mine, one secret wish, that You have not granted me in Your time. I pray more of Your children learn to wait on You for their blessings. Your blessings are abundant, they are streams of living water flowing through deserts. Lord, I pray to keep You first in my heart—and not all

MY BLESSINGS.

And God is able to bless you abundantly, so that in all things
at all times, having all that you need, you will abound in
every good work.

2 Corinthians 9:8 NIV

REMEMBER MY PROMISES

There is so much God has spoken over my life and to me recently, yet I am quick to forget, especially in the moments I need it. The beautiful thing about our Creator is He is always there to remind us of His great love and all the wonderful plans He has for our lives.

Scripture (a.k.a. the Bible) is full of God's promises to humanity, but when you close the door and sit with Him in prayer, you will see how personalized these promises are for your life.

God promises to protect us, fight our battles, give us strength when we are weak, and send His Spirit and wisdom to guide us all our days.

On the days you are filled with doubt and just don't have faith, simply go back to what God said to you. Maybe He spoke through a loving friend or family member, and their words always stuck with you. Whatever it is, remind yourself of it. Write it down! God is full of beautiful promises, and He's not human, so He is able to keep each one without failure.

Dear God, as I write to You today, I recall the beautiful promises You spoke to me in the midst of my pain and suffering. These promises helped get me through the pain and loss. They helped me see past my current circumstances and kept me going. They fueled me on my dark nights and they caused eyes to look to me in wonder . . . how is she? My God, I pray for Your children everywhere, may they hear from You with their ears, may they remember Your promises, and may they know that, regardless of their current circumstance that speaks death over them, they have You to make the way.

You Who has never once failed to deliver on a promise to Your creation because You are the all-powerful God, the beginning and the end. So if You said it, I pray more of us believe it! My God, I pray more of us hear and remember Your personalized promises for our lives. I love You, God, and I love all the beautiful promises You have spoken over me. I love to
REMEMBER MY PROMISES.

He has given us his very great and precious promises.

2 Peter 1:4 NIV

MY PEACE

God wants us to have peace with every step we take. He doesn't want us to just live lives filled with moments of peace. He wants every second to be filled with His peace as long as we are walking in His will.

It's hard to have peace with so many questions, with so much unknown, with responsibilities, pressure, expectations, and so on.

Our Creator did not create us to live in the space of worry. He wants every inch of our lives to be filled with His peace, even in the midst of the unknown.

This is a day-by-day process. A daily surrender to whatever you have zero control over. A daily prayer for God's will to be done in your life. A daily thank-you for all He's done and continues to do.

God is far greater than anything you face in your life, which means He has the power to give you peace at any point. Know that your Creator wants nothing more than for you to enjoy all your days here because it's only for a short amount of time; He is always working on your behalf.

Whatever I tell my 5-year-old niece rings as truth in her eyes. Any fear she had instantly goes away because she knows her aunty V loves her. That's how we are supposed to be each day with God.

You don't have to have peace for tomorrow. Just for today. One day at a time.

Dear God, I pray for more childlike eyes to fill this earth so more people will be like my little niece. They will hear what You say and fear has no choice but to turn away. Lord, I know due to the price You paid with Your Son Who hung on a cross, I know, I truly believe that this has the possibility to be everyone's reality! My God, I pray for Your peace over Your creation, especially those who live far from You. May more of us walk with Your peace. May Your peace be *MY PEACE.*

Rejoice always, pray continually, give thanks in all circumstances;
for this is God's will for you in Christ Jesus.

1 Thessalonians 5:16-18 NIV

✳ *LEAD WITH LOVE* ✳ .

If we knew how much we were loved by God, if we could possibly imagine, we would be more loving to ourselves and others.

Our Creator wants us to lead with love in all areas of our lives because the person you are rude to, the person who is rude to you, is fighting off a lie in their mind about their self-worth. That person is fighting off shame from a choice they made.

In our Creator's eyes, we are His innocent creation. We live in a world 🌍 where people hurt each other. A world where people act from a place of fear and lack of love. A world where people make choices based on greed, lust, and things that don't benefit others. Since we are all connected, due to our actions, everyone becomes more broken.

Lead with love because you never know whose life you are changing. Sometimes it's your life, sometimes it's another person's life, but it's the greatest mission we can ever set our hearts on.

Dear God, I know very well that I do not always lead with love, nor do I always feel love for other people, especially if I am hurt by them. My God, it is easy to love those who are kind to me. How great of a deed is this? Lord, help me, help us lead with love so we can join together and be part of the healing process that so desperately needs to take place in this world. My God, show us, speak to our minds and hearts, help us see what we need to see so we can better

LEAD WITH LOVE.

So in everything, do to others what you would have them do to you, for this sums up the Law and the Prophets.

Matthew 7:12 NIV

I MAKE THE WAY

Oftentimes I want answers, and the minute I don't know and doubt creeps in, instead of bringing it to God in prayer, I am tempted to search for answers elsewhere.

Sweet Vendy, My grace is enough for today
My love is enough for today
My peace is enough for today

Our Creator is our greatest shield. Our best outlet. When you feel emotional or mentally weak, step back into His protective presence.

God will guide us down the best path because He and He alone knows what lies ahead. The hard part is stepping back and letting Him do that.

When you are stressed about the future, you are giving up the blessings of today. Stop robbing yourself. God doesn't like to see His creation worry. I really struggle with this, but when I look back at a major point of distress in my life and reminisce on what little faith I had, I am reminded of how good God is and how I wasted so much time worrying.

Dear Lord, help us hand it all over to You. Please Lord, strengthen our faith because it is You Who makes the way. Help me remember it is not me; never do
I MAKE THE WAY.

Therefore do not worry about tomorrow, for tomorrow will worry about itself. Each day has enough trouble of its own.

Matthew 6:34 NIV

GREAT IS MY FAITHFULNESS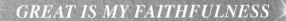

His promise still stands. Great is His faithfulness.

We can be gifted peace and joy in the midst of everything, good or bad, because of what God did. This means, when we suffer, He also allows us to be content. Crazy and truly makes no sense, but I have experienced it personally, so I can testify to this. The most beautiful part is the suffering **NEVER** compares to His blessing, His promise, and His faithfulness.

He moves mountains. He makes ways when there are no ways, and He will do it again and again. Our Creator does the impossible!

He will cover you with his feathers, and under his wings you will find refuge; his faithfulness will be your shield and rampart.

Psalm 91:4 NIV

There is nothing your Creator wouldn't do for you. In His name you will come alive, by His Spirit you will rise. The best part is you do nothing but love, trust, and rest in Him.

T∽H∽A∽N∽K∽♡∽Y∽O∽U

Dear Lord, great are You to me. Under Your wings I have found rest. Your faithfulness has proved to be true, and just as You have said, Your promises come to life time and time again. Great is Your faithfulness. Others may look to my writings one day and never will it be me. Never, no, not I, not mine, never will I be able to say *GREAT IS MY FAITHFULNESS.*

I have faith in God that it will happen just as he told me.

Acts 27:25 NIV

✦ *YOU ARE MINE* ✦

The safest, most peaceful, restful, and best place to be is with God.

The most painful experiences I have ever faced were bearable because of God's love and peace. Our Creator's peace coexists in the most difficult situations . . . it even transcends them.

We will never fully understand certain aspects of life—why horrible things happen to innocent children, for example. But you don't need to fully understand with God. What our Creator offers lifts us up to the point where we don't need to have logical explanations or answers for all aspects of life. All we need to do is trust.

God will always protect you if you allow Him in. He will never let anything happen to you that you can't handle with Him. What will seal this statement as truth is being aware of the decisions and choices you make daily. Some let in sin, which detours you away from His will. Sin is just another word for things outside His will for you. You are not a horrible person if you sin. We all sin due to our flesh, but to stay protected we must choose a life that limits our sin, which is a daily fight and a daily practice.

Dear Lord, thank You for helping me in the battle against sin. I know I will continue to fall short, and my flesh will at times override my spirit that is oh so willing, but I also know greater are You Who dwells in me than he who dwells in this world. I pray to always be Yours and live a life that honors You. I never want You to leave me;

please never leave me! You are my rock, my sweet friend, my
tender heart. It is You Who is so good to me.
YOU ARE MINE.

And the peace of God, which transcends all understanding,
will guard your hearts and your minds in Christ Jesus.

Philippians 4:7 NIV

NEED YOU PLEASE

If God was truly the only One I felt a need to please, everything
would be less complicated and I'd be more happy.

When you are doing what's pleasing to your Creator, not only are
you doing right by yourself, but you are doing right by others as
well. You are the best version of yourself, and there is more to go
around. Your **NO** means no. Your **YES** means yes.

Partnering with God ensures we make wise choices.
He knows everything, including what lies ahead, so
when you feel stressed or torn in certain situations, pray
continuously before you commit or simply send that
text saying yes or no.

Dear Lord, I believe wisdom will be given to me because I have
asked You for her. I have requested that You send her to me to give
me the courage to make certain decisions that have grown me,
caused me to fly. All she births is beauty, bliss, and joy. Her fruits
are bountiful, and in the game of chess, she always wins. Oh, how
I delight in her beauty. But my God, it is You Who brought me to my
knees and because of this, I have requested You to send her to me.
Thank You, my God, for sending her to me. I love what she does in
my life, and I pray You create a need, a desire, in people for more
wisdom. We need more of her and we
NEED YOU, PLEASE.

If any of you lacks wisdom, let him ask God, who gives
generously to all without reproach, and it will be given him.

James 1:5 ESV

I GO BEFORE YOU

Our Creator supports us in our emotions and how we feel. He always thinks of us and watches over everything that concerns us.

Our emotions are always there, but they are not always truthful. I'm learning that acting on my emotions doesn't do much for a situation or me.

Learning how to bring your worries, fears, and emotions to God and leaving them with Him is a skill and process. If you can do this, you instantly have so much peace because you know it will be taken care of and result in the best possible outcome. How is this? You believe the Creator of the universe is going before you.

Dear Lord, my emotions have led me astray, but I no longer fear them or let them dictate my actions. Rather, I acknowledge them and then let them pass. Emotions are from You; You created us to be able to feel. You created us to have free will and choice, and sometimes we partner with our emotions to make choices. My God, I pray that more of us choose to partner with You, Your ways, and not our emotions. Emotions are our friend, they are healthy to have, but they cannot and will not lead us through the wilderness or the dryland. No, it's Your loving-kindness that leads us through the wilderness. It's Your love, Scripture, and promises. It's You Who goes before us. My God, I surrender my emotions to You, take them each time I lay them at Your feet and
I GO BEFORE YOU.

To Him who led His people through the wilderness,
For His lovingkindness endures forever.

Psalm 136:16 AMP

INVITE MY SPIRIT IN

I end up making a mess when I try and do things on my own
by taking matters into my own hands.

Today, God, I ask You to check my heart. I want the place I move
from to honor You. If it doesn't, I ask for Your Spirit to fill me and
lead me, blessing me with the wisdom that stems from a
Spirit-led life.

When we invite our Creator's Spirit in, we are filled
with strength that transcends our emotions and
helps us gracefully navigate all that matters.

Dear Father, I love the fruit of Your Spirit! Will You please send
down love to fill relationships, joy for our days, peace to combat
chaos, forbearance to gift each other, kindness for the moments we
need it the most, goodness that surrounds, faithfulness to lace our
steps, gentleness that leads, and more self-control to protect all we
love. I believe this is possible and will happen when more people
invite in Your Holy Spirit. When we learn what it means and what it
looks like to choose You in both big and small ways. Take more of
us with You. My Lord, my soul belongs to You. I belong to
You, so please take me with You,
INVITE MY SPIRIT IN.

But the fruit of the Spirit is love, joy, peace, forbearance,
kindness, goodness, faithfulness, gentleness and self-control.

Galatians 5:22-23 NIV

MY LOVE

Our Creator's love can get us through anything.

As I reflect this morning, I can't help but feel grateful. Grateful for all the love I have freely received in my life that has shaped my heart. I wouldn't be able to accomplish anything if it weren't for all the love that was poured into me.

> Love is patient, love is kind. It does not envy, it does not boast, it is not proud. . . . It always protects, always trusts, always hopes, always perseveres.
>
> **1 Corinthians 13:4-7 NIV**

Love stays with us. Even when someone is not by your side physically, their actions, words, or the memories you have with them live forever. Once someone pours love into you, they can't take it back. The time has already been given. The encouraging words leave a mark. Some people are better at freely giving love than others. My dad's love was so unconditional and strengthened me in many ways, but my Creator's love is even more remarkable.

God's love is powerful. It defeats death and breathes life. Dead dreams come alive, hope is found, and mountains are moved with your Creator's love.

Dear God, I am amazed by the love You have filled my life with. This love has set me apart; it has protected me. I am chosen and know it because of this love. Growing up, I was always a confident young girl because I had a father who doted on me. He was extremely and uncritically fond of me, praising what felt like my every move. He is now gone, and my confidence, as a result, took a major hit. I have yet to receive this type of adoration from a man, but I am starting to crave it. The good news is I turned to You. Although Al, my beloved father, did a terrific job at loving me, You have exceeded any expectations I could have had, and I am now whole again because of the love I have from You. I still crave it from a man, but only one man, and it will be the one who bends a knee to You, the one from You, because it is You Who protects me with Your love. My God, I pray more women, regardless of the types of fathers they have or don't have, learn to wait on Your love. Because You love so fully, I see my worth and know he must come from You, *MY LOVE.*

Dear friends, let us love one another, for love comes from God.
Everyone who loves has been born of God and knows God.
Whoever does not love does not know God, because
God is love.

1 John 4:7-8 NIV

FOLLOW ME

Our Creator is in charge of the universe. He created it. When we follow His ways, our steps are directed. When His Spirit is with us, we move with wisdom and are protected.

Today is the last day of a chapter in my life, a significant chapter I will always be grateful for. All I can say is, if it weren't for my faith, I would not have lasted. I would not have been able to see the daily blessings, and the door that is open now would not have been there.

When you live with faith, things that normally aren't possible are possible for you—all because God blesses your faith and He is faithful.

One thing I know with all my heart is God's timing is the best, and what He has for you is far better than anything you could ever imagine for yourself.

God, thank You for bringing me this far and for all my blessings. I pray Your will be done.

Dear Lord, it can feel like such a challenge to follow You at times. I see foolish ways appear to win hearts and minds. I see the weak and poor get taken advantage of and the blameless walk through fire or face persecution when standing up for what they know is right. My God, this world is far from You. Its ways are the opposite of Your ways. How do we grow in following You and not in all we see that appears to claim victory? Oh yes, that's it! Meditate, focus, and reflect on You! Day and night, sunrise and sunset, beginnings and endings, new and old, You, You, You! You are the most powerful source there is, and with a snap of Your fingers You can do anything. When I focus on You, I am empowered. I know that I should not grow weary or tired of doing good because all that is good comes from You, Who never changes and remains oh so true to those who walk with You. So today I pray that more souls choose You, and in return we will see, I will see, all that is good begin to

FOLLOW ME.

Every good and perfect gift is from above, coming
down from the Father of the heavenly lights, who
does not change like shifting shadows.

James 1:17 NIV

I FILL

Our Creator fills in the gaps. The lack of love in any relationship, the hurt, the brokenness in any area of our hearts ♡, He has the power to fill.

Your life can be full of loving family members, friends, healthy work relationships, and dreams, but when those things hurt you, He offers never-ending glue that holds you together.

Because we are flawed humans and live in a world 🌍 composed of a lifetime of connected brokenness, no person, dream, career, or relationship will ever fill you the way an all-knowing, perfect God can.

Hurt and injustice will be part of our world, but with God, none of it matters. He is stronger and wiser than anything this world could possibly offer; there's nothing He can't fix or fill.

Dear Lord, let me tell of Your ways, for I have witnessed a filling of brokenness unlike anything this world has ever seen. For there is no telling, no eye has seen, no ear has heard, and no mind has conceived the good You have prepared for the people who love You. I am excited, Father, very excited for all You will do through me and those who learn to choose You! I may still be weak and broken from my loss, but strong like an eagle You promise to make me.

My sweet Vendy, get ready to fly,

You tell me. Yes, an army of angels You will send me, all at Your command they soar and battle in the heavenly sky. Soon the time will wake, deep in my bones I know. Called we all are, choices we all have, and all get to join You in the filling. This world will be filled with light, and a release of healing will break out, by and through You will

I FILL.

He fills my life with good things, so that I stay
young and strong like an eagle. ✘

Psalm 103:5 GNT

YOU BLOSSOM

When a tree or flower blossoms, it produces plenty of fruit or flowers.

When a human blossoms, they develop good, attractive qualities.

To truly be free, awoken, and whole, we must know the darkness of a shadow. It is in that space where the transformation happens. Where the jacket on your heart comes off. Where you can enter a stage of blossoming.

When your Creator holds you and takes care of you, His loving presence causes you to blossom. The beauty in reaching the blossom stage is that you can taste and see the fruits of a divine life and you are filled with so much light.

Dear Lord, You once said to me,

Vendy, I will protect you from this world. I hold you in the palm of My hand, and I will grow you. The protection over your life is so strong, My sweet Vendy. I am doing something through and in you. I created and breathed you to life. Your life was a dream of mine and then I made you. I am always watching you and you must know, My sweet daughter, there is nothing you cannot do.

My God, these words are written on the back of my Bible. You spoke them to me when I was broken. Oh, what these words mean and did for me. My God, thank You for the protection that has covered my life. Thank You for the divine light that grew in the darkest of nights. I am ready and coming back to life, new by Your hand. My God, may many many more of Your sweet daughters and sons blossom. May Your creation know that by Your hand *YOU BLOSSOM.*

The wilderness and the solitary place shall be glad for them;
and the desert shall rejoice, and blossom as the rose.

Isaiah 35:1 KJV

MY FLIGHT

Our Creator enables us to fly. With Him, we soar and fly beyond our wildest dreams. This does not mean there is no turbulence, for it is the turbulence that allows us to transcend all things.

The same way a pilot knows the exact route when navigating through the sky, our Creator knows exactly where He wants to take us—and it's to some unbelievable heights.

When you board an airplane, you don't question the pilot. You have full trust because he is the expert. The same is true with God—He is the expert. His timing could not be more perfect.

So sit back, relax, and enjoy the ride.

Dear Lord, I desperately desire to sit back and enjoy the ride; however, I need Your help. I need You to cast away the anxiety that sneaks up on me, the spinning thoughts, and many what-ifs. Lord, You are my pilot, so teach me how to let go and trust You with each day. For You are the captain of *MY FLIGHT.*

I will instruct you and teach you in the way you should
go; I will counsel you with my loving eye on you.

Psalm 32:8 NIV

JUST THE BEGINNING

I always deliver,
And there is nothing I would not do to bless you,
Protect you,
And guide you

Nothing makes our Creator happier than when we choose Him. His peace, His ways, His love. The wisdom that stems from above not only blesses your life, but those around you, and those to come.

We are all invited to live in our Creator's paradise. Life on earth with His Spirit is filled with endless grace, power, and joy. The waves that come from your Creator bring blessings upon blessings.

Dear Lord, thank You for Your blessings today, tomorrow, and for the ones that are to come. Create in us, God, a heart that can handle the beautiful blessings from You. Through and by Your Holy Son, we are all conquerors if we choose You. Greater and oh so near are You. Please help us see and choose, for with You the best is yet to come. It's *JUST THE BEGINNING.*

Little children, you are from God and have overcome them, for he who is in you is greater than he who is in the world.

1 John 4:4 ESV

✷ *MY WORLD* ✷

The things our Creator wants to show us have no limits, they are
endless and powerful. They are eye-opening, breathtaking,
and truly astonishing.

Our Creator is always with us, looking over us and loving us.
We may not always feel it, but it's true.

Our Creator sometimes keeps encouraging outcomes away from us
as a test. It is not until we learn to fully trust Him, regardless of the
outcome, that we get the desires of our heart. He loves to give the
hoped-for outcome once we have finally learned what it means to
walk by faith.

The greatest blessing to my life is experiencing God's
comfort and wisdom. If it weren't for my loss, I
wouldn't know the depths of God's comfort and
power. Our most painful experiences can be the
keys to unlocking God's world.

There is nothing God wouldn't do for us. On your grief-filled nights,
just remember that a purified heart accompanies your suffering, one
that learns how to see and hear from God. Now tell me, what could
be more powerful than this?

Dear Lord, comfort all Your children who mourn. Then, once
they learn what it means to walk by faith and not by sight,
please bless them. Bless them beyond belief, bless them in a
way that turns this world upside down and causes all those around

them to look up! Thank You, Lord, for handing us, the suffering souls, the keys to unlocking Your world. The view I now have is from above. I see the world oh so differently, and I love how You have changed
MY WORLD.

Blessed are those who mourn, for they will be comforted.

Matthew 5:4 NIV

SEPTEMBER

NEW HEIGHTS

Our Creator loves to see us reach new heights in life. The view from the top is what keeps many people going, but as we climb our mountain 🏔, it's important to reflect.

True reflection allows you to see how far you have come, how far God has brought you, and it fills you with hope. It shows you that He did it once and will continue to do it in new and more profound ways.

Know God is able to infuse the most challenging hike, the steepest climb, with joy and peace. Joy and peace so mighty that they transcend the understanding of the human mind.

Remember you are never alone; you are loved and you have a God Who is excited to climb the mountain with you. Take a moment to sit and enjoy the view with Him today.

Dear Lord, I love the melody You play for me while I climb to the mountaintops. The tunes in my life, because they are from You, keep me going with a pep in my step. Yes, I dance to the beat, sway my hips, and move to Your sweet melody. I giggle at what is to come when my heart feels heavy because I know it's You Who I hand full control over to. Yes, it's You that brings me to *NEW HEIGHTS.*

The Sovereign LORD is my strength; he makes my feet like the feet of a deer, he enables me to tread on the heights. For the director of music. On my stringed instruments.

Habakkuk 3:19 NIV

MY ROADMAP

Our Creator has the roadmap. He knows exactly how to navigate this complex world and feeds our spirits so we can win daily battles.

His roadmap doesn't always look the way we want it to, but the minute you let go of how you want it to look and simply trust Him, He grants you the deepest desires of your heart ♡ . . . even ones you didn't know you wanted.

God placed those desires in your heart, and He is the only one that can continually feed you what you need to eventually land you where you desire to be.

When you reach a dead end by doing it your way, invite God in. He will send His Spirit, and by His side you will travel far and wide. What He has to offer is greater than any dream and any human being.

The roadmap our Creator has for each person is different, so we each must seek Him. Only He knows the right formula to feed your soul and bless you with the best possible outcome for your life.

Dear God, You have given me the secret recipe. To win my battles each day, I must praise You, that way Your name and all You do grows greater than the discouragement that lies before me.

Then I must seek You daily and invite Your Spirit in. With this comes wisdom and specific instructions that keep me on Your path, so I can follow
MY ROADMAP.

I will instruct you and teach you in the way you should go; I will counsel you with my loving eye on you.

Psalm 32:8 NIV

MY DOOR

God loves to see us filled with joy. He loves to see us thrive. We go through difficulties in life, but on the other side there is a rainbow waiting for us. It's just a matter of making it through the rain.

God doesn't bless us with anything we cannot handle. When we trust, He opens the **RIGHT** doors just in time. It may be a struggle getting there, but when the door is from Him, you will be ready.

No matter what lies ahead, know that all things are possible with your Creator. You may not feel energized, powerful, or ready, but with a God that goes before you, there is nothing you cannot do.

We must put any shortcomings we have in His hands and believe He will do the rest. He brought you this far and wants nothing more than to make the way for you! There is so much strength and protection He gives on a daily basis that we are so unaware of.

His power is sufficient for all situations. Whatever lies ahead, any fears or doubts, bring them to your Creator and He will make the way.

Dear Lord, I love Your rainbows. When they appear, the sun is usually to follow along with a clear sky. My God, I am even learning to enjoy the rain that comes before the rainbow. You have grown my faith in the rain, and now I know the pouring doesn't last forever;

when the rainbow does come, I can appreciate it more. I can take in the colors and beauty with open eyes. So please continue to teach me and all Your creation what it looks like to dance in the rain. Show us that the rain should not bring shame, but rather strength, which makes us sufficient for all different types of climates. My God, I pray for more of Your timing in my life so I can walk on paths only from You. May You continue to direct my every step and open *MY DOOR*.

At the right time, I, the LORD, will make it happen.

Isaiah 60:22 NLT

REMEMBER MY WORDS

Vendy, I will enable you, strengthen you, and equip you
All you have to do is focus on leading with love
and putting My ways first
Success and protection will flow from this
My words are powerful
They move and have supernatural strength
So repeat them to yourself and reflect in moments
of doubt or when lies creep in

Persevere in placing your hope in God's love and power.
This is a daily task; checking back in with what God
says about His creation makes all the difference. Moment
to moment, whenever you need it, look to Him. Our Creator
is always with us, watching and making the way.

Dear Father, I know I need Your strength for all that is next. I know
I will not be able to make it through if You are not directing my each
move. Lord, please show me the way. When I let fear overrule, cast
it away. Signal me to sound Your praise so I persevere in this game!
Give me peace, not the peace this world speaks, but true peace that
transcends situations and circumstances. Yes, that's it, that's what
I need. And when I make it through the day, may I look up to You
with gratitude. Please Father, hear my prayer and
REMEMBER MY WORDS.

Now may the Lord of peace himself give you peace at
all times and in every way. The Lord be with all of you.

2 Thessalonians 3:16 NIV

MULTIPLY OUR MOMENTS

Vendy, I am your greatest resource
I press pause on the world 🌎
And I give you peace in exchange for whatever
short amount of time you give me
I do what no human being can do

🔑 Our Creator has the power to be our peace.
What He has to offer, no one else can offer.

Dear God, thank You for today and for giving me peace in the moments I choose You. I ask that You continue to multiple our moments so Your Spirit can perform in me what is not humanly possible otherwise. 🙏 🤍 Lord, if You do this for me, I know I can make it through. Please help me bring Your gracious loving-kindness and divine approval so I can make it through. My God, please continue to
MULTIPLY OUR MOMENTS.

The Lord make His face shine upon you [with favor], And be gracious to you [surrounding you with lovingkindness]; The Lord lift up His countenance (face) upon you [with divine approval], And give you peace [a tranquil heart and life].

Numbers 6:25-26 AMP

DIVINE LOVE

Our Creator offers divine love. It's so overwhelming and good, we as humans are not used to it. When I enter into prayer and ask God about certain things, His replies leave me baffled at times.

Today try to be present and grateful. All the good, bad, and beautiful things that are happening in your life serve a much greater purpose with your Creator. So take it all in.

The good marks His power and love. The bad, when accepted with courage, is an opportunity to receive God's grace, be filled, and grow so you will be ready for much larger blessings.

Dear God, I love Your ability to perplex me. Just when I think I have it figured out, You have a way of flipping things inside out and upside down. The beauty in this stems from Your love. Because we live in a world that dwells far from You, I know the confusion will always rest in my flesh. The horrible, heartbreaking things we see may cast discouragement over our hearts and minds, but because of You we are able to overcome. Conquerors we are. A conqueror I now am through your
DIVINE LOVE.

No, in all these things we are more than conquerors through him who loved us.

Romans 8:37 NIV

✦ *I QUALIFY* ✦

Anything you want, you can have
Anything you dream of is yours
As long as it's My time, My will, and My price
All you need is Me, sweet V

We are so much stronger than we know. With God, we can do more than we are capable of on our own. I promise, much of the pain you have experienced has prepared you for what is next.

All you have walked through will one day act as your strength and no longer your crutch. Remember Who got you through and remember God strengthens you.

Anything you want, you can have, as long as it's in His good will for you. Make your needs known to God and He will do the rest. It doesn't matter what may be working against you. Put your trust in your Creator, fight the limiting thoughts, and acknowledge how powerful and mighty your God is. He will do it all: direct your path, go before you, and equip you. 🤍

Dear Lord, I cannot testify enough to Your power and might that was placed on display in my life when I was in distress. It was there, in the cold wilderness and desert land, where I grew into something new. Divine, even! Now as I venture on new grounds, there are still broken parts of me that need filling, that need much of You, but it will all be okay. This I know because I hold the keys that will get me through. It's time with You. Yes, that's it, that's all each of us

will ever need. Time with You gives us what we need for all that
is next. So I am ready, enlarged through my distress,
I QUALIFY.

Thou hast enlarged me when I was in distress.

Psalm 4:1 KJV

LIFE WITH ME

Our Creator has a way of deepening our souls, our existences, and through this process a strong desire for more truth is created. By His hand, we then crave ways filled with wisdom because they're rich and produce fruit.

When our souls grow in spiritual maturity, we are exposed more and more to our Creator's ways, His profound secrets. God trusts us with greater power.

The heavens are higher than the earth. Our Creator's thoughts and ways are higher than our own.

Limiting God, trying to make His ways predictable so we can understand, does us no good.

Dear Lord, I really need Your help trusting. Trusting in You and not all I see. Trusting that it is You Who will fight my battles, move on my behalf, and honor me! I want to be a soul that You trust to fill with power and truths, prophecy, and gifts from above, because of the way I have learned to lean on You, bend a knee, and seek You. I know oftentimes I do not fully understand Your ways, but I do trust that You will never lead me astray. I love this new life I have, one that dwells extra close to You. Please keep me close, and when I turn away from You, forgive me. The heavens are just so much higher and closer to You, and this fallen earth is sometimes so hard for me, but I know now that all I need to do is trust You with all my heart

to make it through. I know the life You desire to create for me
is much greater than anything I could ever come up with.
So, Father, please always do
LIFE WITH ME.

Trust in the Lord with all your heart and lean
not on your own understanding.

Proverbs 3:5 NIV

* *MY SWING* *

It doesn't matter what your age is, in our Creator's eyes, we are all small children, and because of this He desires to give You a view that will help You make it through. Today He placed me on a swing set overlooking the earth. I watched my family and friends move about their days and saw my coworkers in motion.

God gives us elevated views so we can see the things that cause us stress and realize how small they are in comparison to where He stands.

The disappointments in life are not intended to weigh you down forever, but rather bring you closer to a loving Creator Who sees all things and works them out for your best interest.

When God is the constant in your life, He provides stability and direction in unpredictable environments. Just as young children do not worry when they are by their parent's side, neither should you. 🤍 He just wants you to enjoy the view.

Dear Lord, thank You for placing me on Your swing and giving me a view from above. Although I am not ready to let go of my morning matcha, close my journal, and get ready for the workday ahead, I will because of the view You gave me. After sitting with You, I realized the stress weighing heavy on my tiny heart not only hurts You, but I was never designed to carry it in the first place. I am not equipped on my own. But You continue to show me that You are always by my side, my constant companion. Even when I sleep, You so tenderly watch over me. My God, I pray for all Your

children today who battle stress and anxiety, please give them direction in their unpredictable situations and make room for them on
MY SWING.

I lift up my eyes to the mountains—where does my help come from? My help comes from the LORD, the Maker of heaven and earth. He will not let your foot slip—he who watches over you will not slumber.

Psalm 121:1-3 NIV

MY DESIRE

My sweet Vendy, I designed you
to be carefree, free from anxiety
I designed you to be loving and full of life

As we go through life, this world puts chains on us. We are bound by fear and future worries that stem from our thoughts. ☁ Both current and future worries exist in our minds and cause stress!

Focus on Me and the mystical ways I move
One task at a time
This will restore your energy and
make you more effective
This will bring joy in the midst of your hustle
This will allow you to be My child
I will restore you back to the carefree and loving nature
I designed you to live in
I promise to make the way and do the rest

Our Creator wants nothing more than to reset and restore us to our original disposition. We were designed to know and have His peace. Unfortunately, we live in a fallen world 🌍 where that seems impossible at times; however, God says He will give us joyful spirits in the middle of our struggle.

🔑 God has a way of using everything for your advancement and growth. He is sovereign, and if your Creator says He will bless your mind with peace regardless of how stressful your situation may be, then He will do it. 🙏 ♡ Dear God, I ask for a grateful heart and to receive all You have put in front of me with a joyful spirit because I know the things that cause me stress lead me to You and grow me. They teach me how to have joy no matter what I face. They teach me the power of praise and positivity over complaints. May You honor all Your children who turn to You and cling to Your ways. May You bless all Your children who dwell far from You with this truth. May more of Your children pave the way with Your praise. May Your children sing of Your faithfulness through generations, for it is Your love and Your hand that causes them to endure. Break chains and purify hearts so more can walk in their desires that help set others free, for this, my Lord, is *MY DESIRE.*

Enter his gates with thanksgiving and his courts with praise; give thanks to him and praise his name. For the LORD is good and his love endures forever; his faithfulness continues through all generations.

Psalm 100:4-5 NIV

MY PRESENCE

You have been there loving me and helping me.
You give me whatever wisdom I may have.
You have always taken care of me. My heart 🤍 and my soul follow
close behind You, my dear God.
I rest on Your clouds. ☁️

When we create a safe space and practice bringing things to
our Creator, we find rest, encouragement, and strength.

When we are aware of how great our God is, we know He
never drops the ball and carries us through all things.
When we grow in relationship with Him and He dwells
in us, we become godly and He empowers us to do
anything we set our minds to.

Dear God, today I ask that Your Holy Spirit opens my eyes to **ALL**
the ways You are looking out and moving. When I am aware of You
and Your power over every challenging situation that may arise in
my daily life, I am equipped to face all that lies ahead. I really love
You so much. I don't think I have ever experienced a love like this.
I pray my soul always follows close behind You. Please never leave
my side, and show others, more people young and old, what it is like
to live a life close to the divine. Please Lord, join me today as
I drive, as I work, as I eat, play, and rest. Please never leave
MY PRESENCE.

When I remember You on my bed, I meditate on You in the night watches.
Because You have been my help. Therefore in the shadow of Your wings I
will rejoice. My soul follows close behind You; Your right hand upholds me.

Psalm 63:6-8 NKJV

✳ *SEE ME*

So often we go through our days and see only the things that cause us stress. We let them eat at us and forget the blessings.

Choose to see the good. Nothing in life will ever be perfect, but when you are grateful for what you have and take care of it, your Creator will bless you with more. ♡ No matter the challenge you face each day, set aside moments to enjoy the wonderful scenery in your life. Maybe it's a call from a loved one, an encouraging text from a friend, or the bliss that accompanies a sunset.

Dear Lord, help me to view my life as a training session. The steeper the mountain 🏔, the greater Your adventure. Don't let me lose sight of the daily blessings during my climb. My God, I am learning the more I am able to see You, fix my eyes on You, the better my climb! Father, in this season I believe You are teaching me that it will always be You at my side. No matter the love that enters and leaves my life, as long as I have You, the possibility to be filled with delight is mine. Please Father, never leave me.
I pray You always watch over and
SEE ME.

Then I was constantly at his side. I was filled with delight
day after day, rejoicing always in his presence.
Proverbs 8:30 NIV

✦ YOUR LIFE . . . I WRITE ✦

When we believe our Creator, the One Who created the strongest forces in this world, like love 🤍 and the vast ocean 🌊 , is the writer of our lives, we find rest. We find rest even when we are carrying a heavy cross because we know it's all part of the story, the greater picture.

🗝 Lift your heavy cross with a patient spirit and a smile, and then with no complaints just move. When we do this, in time, we will see how the cross is what grew us and pushed us up the mountain, not what caused us to stumble.

🗝 If you allow your Creator to write your life, you have peace in the middle of confusion and doubt. You are strengthened. If you knock, He will open the right door for you.

It's easy to forget that God is always in charge. He is especially close to those who need Him most, to those who need comfort for their souls. He will lift you up and guide you exactly where you are supposed to be. There are no limits to what He can do. The only limits are the ones that exist in our minds. Even then, if we turn to our Creator, He has the power to destroy them.

Dear Lord, as I have grown to know You more intimately, I know You are a very intentional God. I know You do not make mistakes because You are not human. I know You have created me for a special purpose and placed me on this earth, knowing every detail of my life before I do. My God, I know You to be meticulous, showing great attention to detail. You are very careful and precise even in the words You speak to me, knowing exactly what my heart needs and where my every thought will lead. So today I have one prayer and one request, and it's that You write more of Your children's lives. Yes, we must choose You in order for You to take our pens, but Father, please, we want lives that reflect more of the divine, more light so the darkness will flee! My God, we all have a purpose, we just need Your help. We need You to write each chapter. Oh, publisher of my peace, I love when You speak to me . . .

Sweet V,
YOUR LIFE . . . I WRITE.

And we know that in all things God works for the good of those who love him, who have been called according to his purpose.

Romans 8:28 NIV

I WRAP MY ARMS

Around you

Hold on to Me as you go through your day today
Moment by moment, think of Me,
walk with Me, lean on Me
I'm always here, wherever you go, Vendy

When God is your confidence, He will go before you.

Dear Lord, I so greatly need You to intercede on my behalf. I so easily grow weak when I think all You have called me to do is all on me. I lose confidence because I can't do it, I just can't do it without You. But I am learning that is the point. You did not create us to do mighty things without You. No, that's what makes them oh so mighty. It's the Holy Spirit that moves in and fills the space in broken people, who then go on to accomplish wonderful things. Things that point to the heavens and bring about good. Please, Father, wrap Your heavenly arms around me. I need You to hold me really close, and as You do, around You
I WRAP MY ARMS.

Therefore he is able to save completely those who come to God through him, because he always lives to intercede for them.

Hebrews 7:25 NIV

LOOK TO ME

Look to Me in your weakness,
Look to Me in your fullness
Look to Me always because I have just what you need
And there are things that only I can give you

When we look to God in all things, the good and the
bad, we see them in a new light. When we look to
Him when times are good, we are aware and our
Creator fills us with gratitude. When we look to
Him when times are bad, He gives us hope
and strengthens us. 🖤

Dear God, in my weakness I turn to You. I run to You. In my
fullness, I must learn to keep looking to You. I am tempted when
I am full to do things on my own because I have the energy,
excitement, and feel oh so good, but how could anything ever make
me full without You? Yes, I have reached a point in my life where
after the breaking, crushing, and pressing, the new wine in me craves
what brings honor first to You. Because without You, my foundation
is weak. I pray more seek Your face always because there are things
our souls need that only You can give. May I forever and always
look to You. My ways have only led me astray, no longer will I
LOOK TO ME.

Look to the LORD and his strength; seek his face always.

1 Chronicles 16:11 NIV

MY WATERS

The ocean's depth and beauty are signs of God's handiwork. Examples of His pure and wonderful creation placed on earth for us to enjoy.

My sweet child,
life is a series of rough and calm waters
The beauty is knowing that I am by your side,
with you in both
You will have calm days, you will have busy days
You will have joyful days, you will have pain-filled days
There is beauty in both because
I am always at your side

God is in control of the waves that surround you.

When you are in the ocean, swimming through life,
I am in control of the waters
The ocean was not created by man, but Me
I will bring you through high tides and low tides
Your time with Me is never wasted
Your time with Me is what feeds you 🤍

Dear Lord, the amount of time we spend with You is critical. The shape of my heart is molded by Your all-knowing hand. Like the rocks that line the coast, the more exposed my heart is to You, the deeper the impression on my heart. The mornings mark my favorite time of day with You. I love to wake with You because

You know just what I need to hear. You know the thoughts that
will enter my mind before they enter my mind. You have a way
of soothing me and preparing me for the day ahead. You show me
the way I need to go with a timeline I can trust because I choose to
belong to You. With the rising and falling of the sea, remind me that
You have the power over the moon and sun, controlling the tides as
they roll in. Please remind me it is You that stills

MY WATERS.

Let the morning bring me word of your unfailing love, for
I have put my trust in you. Show me the way I should go,
for to you I entrust my life.

Psalm 143:8 NIV

I REVEAL

I know that nothing I dream of or work for will compare to God's plan for my life. My prayer of surrender and thanks is to be used by God in whatever way He designed me.

I pray my life will be a story You create with Your hands. I pray a stroke of Your art, vision, and master creation be reflected in me.

May Your Spirit dwell in all who praise You and love You. Please direct our every word and every move.

Dear God, I see Your timeline. I see what a beautiful life You are creating. I ask that my life be a dedication to You and the power of Your love. I pray every hour, minute, and second be dedicated to You. I know You will use my current sufferings and they will not compare to the glory that, by and through You,

I REVEAL.

I consider that our present sufferings are not worth comparing with
the glory that will be revealed in us.

Romans 8:18 NIV

MY WHIRLWIND

We want change, we are ready for change . . . until it comes.

Our Creator takes us to new heights. The journey is testing, and there will be days where you question everything you once found peace in. There will be days where nothing seems to make sense.

Look to Me

Giving thanks to God opens paths that transcend your understanding. He is in charge of the whirlwind that is about to take place in your life. And the only way to truly enjoy your life in the midst of the madness is to find peace and comfort in God's sovereignty. God's truth. God's pure goodness that will guide your every step.

Dear God, this next chapter is what I have asked You for, but now I am starting to think I am not ready, nor do I really know what I want. I think I know, then it comes and I begin to question. But I guess that's part of the process, and sometimes You have to let us walk through certain things so we know for ourselves and never have to question or play with the what-ifs. Lord, I pray for the hearts and minds all over the world that are entering a new season, a new chapter. May You fill them, strengthen them, and bless them with wisdom for all that lies ahead. I know, without You there is no getting through MY WHIRLWIND.

For the LORD is good and his love endures forever; his faithfulness continues through all generations.

Psalm 100:5 NIV

LIFE FROM ABOVE

With Me there are no worries
You are right where you are supposed to be, sweet Vendy
I hold you high above, your feet dangle in the sky
You see this world 🌎 from the clouds ☁️ , and
you should be filled with fear
You are just floating in the sky, but I am holding you,
I am giving you this breathtaking view
And because it is Me that's holding you,
you have no fear
You know you are right where you're supposed to be
You take in the view and you are in amazement
You don't know how you got there, there is no logical
explanation for it aside from Me

This is what our Creator does: He takes us places we can't
go on our own. He shows us how beautiful and
fast our lives move, how time flies. All He wants is for
us to be close to Him so we can enjoy the view.

God enables us to see things from His view, not the world's
view. 🌎 He simply removes human limitations and
fills us with divine encounters.

Dear Lord, where is it I can go that You do not see me? Can I ever
hide from You? My God, I know You will lead me to new grounds,
ones that should scare me due to the view. But I take heart;

because I have You, I will be able to take in the breathtaking view.
I will see the limitations placed on me and laugh as the divine
encounters begin to fill my life. I will continue to reach because it
is You Who enables my view and fills my
LIFE FROM ABOVE.

And when I am lifted up from the earth,
I will draw everyone to myself.

John 12:32 NLT

MY GOD

New Wine. 🍷 New Ground.

Make me Your vessel. Make me whatever You want me to be and in me will be new power, new freedom. I will lay down my own flames so I can carry Your new fire today. 🎶

🗝️ In the crushing and pressing, I surrender.

Dear God, I ask to be used by You. I ask to be Your vessel. I ask You to transform me into whatever You want me to be. I thank You, I am forever grateful for the crushing. It was through the crushing where I found life in You, life and hope that does not compare to anything this world could offer. 🤍🙏 So with this new life, I pray to give it all to You. The crushing and pressing made new wine and it's more divine. It is filled with notes I could have never achieved on my own. May You pair it with just the right things, for I am Yours,

MY GOD.

Even to your old age and gray hairs I am he, I am he who will sustain you. I have made you and I will carry you; I will sustain you and I will rescue you.

Isaiah 46:4 NIV

TENDERIZE MY HEART

When you tenderize food, you slowly cook it. It's a process that takes time.

Life will never be fair, but that doesn't mean you shouldn't be. We all experience hurt and pain from other people, but if you ask God to use it and surrender it to Him, He will turn that hurt into strength. He will place purpose over that hurt so it doesn't move on to another person, but ends with you.

You are protected, strong, and God goes before you. Stay true to your heart when it comes to people, and do by them only what you'd like for yourself. You may not see the fruits of this overnight, but you will begin to see how God honors you. Trust me when I say it leaves others confused!

Dear God, I ask You to tenderize my heart. I ask that You take all hurtful situations or feelings I experience over the course of my life and use them to teach me compassion. And when it's time for me to move and make decisions due to the authority You have placed over my life, I will act with a tender heart. So, my God, even though it hurts, continue to

TENDERIZE MY HEART.

Since God chose you to be the holy people he loves, you must clothe yourselves with tenderhearted mercy, kindness, humility, gentleness, and patience. Make allowance for each other's faults, and forgive anyone who offends you.

Colossians 3:12-13 NLT

ONLY I CAN DO

There are certain blessings in your life, in my life, that came from God and could have only been from our Creator.

We are able to walk through certain doors because He blesses us with courage, grace, and His timing.

God takes hold of each day if we give it to Him.
He reminds us that we don't handle things
alone, and He empowers us so we can move
forward, capable and equipped, to do all things.

Dear God, thank You for doing more than I could possibly imagine in my life. I pray Your Spirit continues to feed me in my moments of need. I know there are certain things that only You can do. Father, please equip more of Your children. We want to see a move by and through You. I know, Father, we all have a unique set of gifts and we are all called, but not all follow. Empower me to do what is possible with You, whatever it is You are calling me to do.
Please show me what
ONLY I CAN DO.

Now to him who is able to do immeasurably more than all we ask
or imagine, according to his power that is at work within us.

Ephesians 3:20 NIV

DEEPEN MY LOVE

The stronger my desire to know God more intimately, the more joy I have, and the more my perspective in life shifts.

I can do more, live more, and experience more because my lifeline to the heavens is lifting me. Lifting me above so I can see things from new heights and hear God more clearly.

When God is the strongest desire in our lives, we begin to choose Him daily. When we choose Him, we are choosing a fruitful life that changes this world. A life that gives life to others. A life filled with fruits of His Spirit. A life filled with life from above.

Dear Lord, as my love grows for You, so does my desire to see justice. And as my desire for justice grows, so does my will to honor You. And as my will to honor You grows, the opportunities grow to do just that. Father, continue to expand hearts all over the world; may they continue to grow in love for You, resulting in ruling authorities that honor and change the world. You already sent one Man Who changed the world by moving in the hearts and minds of believers everywhere. Father, continue to move in my heart and Your believers' hearts everywhere. Father, please keep it going.

DEEPEN MY LOVE.

For this very reason, make every effort to add to your faith goodness; and to goodness, knowledge; and to knowledge, self-control; and to self-control, perseverance; and to perseverance, godliness; and to godliness, mutual affection; and to mutual affection, love.

2 Peter 1:5-7 NIV

CONFIDENCE LIES IN ME

When your Creator reveals powerful things to you, it's hard to turn away. Yes, things may happen in your life that do not confirm these promises in the moment, but there is always a divine timeline at play.

Keep going, striving, and persevering because you have faith in an unfailing God, not because you do things by your own limited human mind.

Your words, actions, and life matter. Everything you do matters. What you speak over yourself and others influences your physical and emotional well-being.

Whatever areas of your life you need help in, call on God and watch as you move forward with strength and confidence.

Dear Lord, these new waters are challenging to navigate. My confidence has taken a hit since the passing of my dad. My energy and zest for life have changed overnight, and I am not sure of the deep waters I am currently swimming through. I have been tempted to turn parts of me to the attention of a man, one that is not from You, but for whatever reason . . . I continue to choose You. I know there is no quick fix for what You would like me to do or learn from all of this, and I know You to be very faithful to me and will only test me with what I can handle. So, Father, continue to provide a way and create in me an enduring heart that scares the enemy! May his knees lock and legs turn to spaghetti. May the greatest tempter there is now flee when he sees me. I pray for strength beyond belief, and not just for me, but for all Your women and men that seek You. Now Your

CONFIDENCE LIES IN ME.

No temptation has overtaken you except what is common to mankind. And God is faithful; he will not let you be tempted beyond what you can bear. But when you are tempted, he will also provide a way out so that you can endure it.

1 Corinthians 10:13 NIV

I GUIDE

I am always amazed at the depth and wisdom of God. His answers are simple and pure, yet I never seem to arrive there on my own.

You know you are where your Creator wants you to be in life when you are learning and growing with every step.

You know you are where your Creator wants you to be when you don't really have the time, but you make it for Him because you know how much of His guidance you need.

God has a unique way of guiding each of us through life. It is usually in the challenging situations where our Creator uncovers our gifts and develops us. Only He knows what it takes to make each of us bend a knee.

God's Spirit feeds our souls, and He creates conquerors in us. We overcome adversity and grow stronger with every battle. The fruits of adversity produce peace in any and all situations. They produce healing and hope for people in your life and people around the world.

Dear Lord, it's hard to picture where my life will end, nor do I usually think that far into the future. But I imagine I will be an old lady whose skin hangs and whose bones are thinned. My hair will be white and my eyes not so bright. But, Father, I know I will still have You. I know You are the only One I will always have. Father, when it's all said and done and I make it to the end, may You say, *Sweet Vendela, job well done.*

Yes, this will bring delight to my ears because I have fought the good fight for the One Who was always by my side. In my old age, Father, I want to say it was all for You and by Your grace that I learned to bend a knee to You—and it didn't take my entire existence to get me there. I want to say thank You, God, for being my eternal guide. Because You dwell in me, empowered I walk and
Your baby lambs
I GUIDE.

For this God is our God for ever and ever;
he will be our guide even to the end.

Psalm 48:14 NIV

OCTOBER

ENOUGH FOR EVERYONE

Find rest in Me so you can do more, more than anything you
could have ever imagined
I calm the storm or sometimes I place you in the middle
Then gently whisper the solution into your ear
I hold your hand and walk you through the day, and
as you move, you gift others with My Spirit

When you seek rest with God, you recharge in
ways that no amount of sleep or worldly
resources could ever supply.

When you find rest in Me,
there is enough love in you to go around
So everyone feels My presence

Dear Lord, if only I would have known what I was praying for when
I asked You to use me! A pure heart You create, but with much pain.
A steadfast, enduring spirit I have, but the fire almost burned me!
My Lord, You have placed me in the middle of the storm, and You
do not plan on calming it, but rather whispering to me the solution.
The problem is I can't seem to be still for long enough to hear it, and
it's surrounding me. Father, I can't be still for long enough because
I have no time to be still. You must know I need to sleep! My God,
I am barely enough for myself today. How can I possibly be enough
for everyone? What's that? . . . Pray? Pray to You wherever my feet
lead? Pray to You when I am driving, when I am at my desk, eating,
drinking my coffee, walking, and rushing. Pray to You during these

things? I don't have to be in my room in my cozy pj's? Ohhhh okay,
I will try this, but Your whisper is so gentle, will I be able to hear
You? I should just step away, even for a moment throughout my
day . . . Yes, I will try this. For today I need so much of You, so
I will do just this. I will pray pray pray, that way today I can be
ENOUGH FOR EVERYONE.

Create in me a pure heart, O God, and
renew a steadfast spirit within me.

Psalm 51:10 NIV

TRUST

Trust is a powerful action. To trust is to hold a firm belief in the reliability, truth, ability, or strength of someone or something.

 When we trust one another, in relationships of all sorts, we create an atmosphere of peace.

Dear God, help me trust You today. Help me trust that You are taking care of me, filling in the gaps of my many shortcomings. Help me trust that You are guiding me throughout my journey of life. Father, I am learning a lack of trust in any relationship results in a lack of peace. When we grow in trust, we grow in peace. Father, I am a friend, sister, daughter, granddaughter, coworker, and aunty. As my life evolves, I may one day add mother and wife to this very lovely list. I am finding with the current relationships I have that trust lays the foundation for love. How do we love if we do not trust? My God, I know it brings deep joy to Your heart when I trust You. When things bother me and eat at my thoughts, You love it when I lay them at Your feet and trust You. When I am able to do this, I receive peace! So how can I purely love if I have no trust in myself? I cannot give peace, nor can I receive it, without trust. Father, help Your lambs learn what it means to *TRUST.*

But I trust in you, LORD; I say, "You are my God."

Psalm 31:14 NIV

STRENGTHEN ME

When my heart is heavy and full and I just don't know what
to do, I find strength in You.

Ask the Lord to lead the way. ♡

Dear God, help me place my hope in You all day long, especially
on the days I need more rest and I am confused. I need Your
presence on this journey of life all my days to enjoy it, because I
now feel so empty without You. If I learn to keep You first in my
heart, You will make my path like the morning sun — bright and
life-giving. God, comfort my bruised heart, restore my vision and
love for life, fill me with Your Spirit, and strengthen me so other
bruised hearts will have hope for their days. Make the way, show
me with every breath I take, hold me close, and
STRENGTHEN ME.

The path of the righteous is like the morning sun, shining
ever brighter till the full light of day.

Proverbs 4:18 NIV

✴ ONLY ME ✴

I will restore what only I can restore
I will heal what only I can heal
I will bring together what only I can bring together

The more time I spend with God, the more time I can reflect and see His divine timeline at play in my life. It's so divine, so powerful; it's nothing I could have ever created or done on my own.

Your Creator is omnipresent, which means He does not operate under the rules and constraints of time. He is present everywhere at the same time. This means His meticulous plan for your life is already done. Due to this, He wants us to be present, never to worry, and to enjoy every moment of our short time here.

Of course, this is much easier said than done, but God loves when we cast our worries onto Him because He can see us grow lighter and the light within us grow brighter. 💡

Dear Lord, I know we each have free will; therefore, Your will might not always be done on earth. With that said, I also know You are omnipotent, You have unlimited power, and are able to do anything, which means even when things happen on earth that are **NOT** according to Your good will, You remain all-powerful and can weave together a plan better than the first! I pray to You today requesting that You release Your children from worry. We all have reasons that cause us to worry in our lives, but the closer we grow to the omnipotent Creator, the less territory worry takes. Father, You see my every coming and every going, You know my every thought, so please do what only You can do in my life. Restore what only You can restore, heal what only You can heal, and bring together what only You can bring together. Orchestrate it all! My Lord, please do right by Your children so people can see, hear, and testify that it could have only been by the omnipotent God. May You be able to say it was

ONLY ME.

The LORD watches over you—the LORD is your shade at your right hand; the sun will not harm you by day, nor the moon by night. The LORD will keep you from all harm—he will watch over your life; the LORD will watch over your coming and going both now and forevermore.

Psalm 121:5-8 NIV

EXHALE LIFE

I breathe life into the scars of your heart, Vendy 🤍

God has the ability to breathe into our scars and give them life. He takes a big inhale and gently blows His breath over your heart. The scars heal and the skin covering your heart is now stronger and more flexible. The blood in your heart is more vibrant.

Ask God what scars are on your heart. Then, take the time and invite Him in; ask Him to breathe life into your scars.

Dear God, today I ask for Your grace. I will need enough for myself and some extra to give to others. I am learning to love the scars on my heart because they create in me resilient, yet more forgiving skin. Pumping in my heart is a deeper red that shines through. My Lord, I love You and I pray You write every chapter of my life. Thank You for breathing life into my scars. 🙏 May You use each of them for Your greater good. May they

EXHALE LIFE!

The Spirit of God has made me; the breath of the Almighty gives me life.

Job 33:4 NIV

MORE OF ME

God help me see. Open my eyes, help me be grateful, fill me with
Your love and joy. Help me focus on You. Pull back the curtains and
give me understanding. Shine a light 💡 where I need it. Replace my
worry with gratitude. Fill me with Your Spirit. Please, I need
more of You.

The answer is You. No amount of sleep, work,
preparation, or relaxation will do for me what
only You can do. I ask today for more of You. 🤍

Dear Lord, I am burning the candle at both ends, and my body and
mind are growing weak. It is causing me to be weary and I feel
burdened. This was **NEVER** me. I know You allow certain things
to happen, and in this season I will need to cling to You to make it
through. Not only is my flesh weak, but I lack understanding and
insight. I need more than rest for my body, I need You to give my
mind rest. You see, I have never been an anxious person. My entire
life I have been the opposite . . . oh so carefree! But those days feel
long gone; I am in a desolate land. Father, I need rest for my body
and mind. I need more of You to combat the anxiety, for my heart is
crushed in mighty ways. Stress now follows me into each new day.
This I know is not from You, but I know it is there for me so I can
learn to pick up the key that unlocks my peace. Yet, for me to pick
up the key, I know it will take more of You and not
MORE OF ME.

Come to me, all you who are weary and
burdened and I will give you rest.

Matthew 11:28 NIV

I AM YOURS

We, as humans, have limitations. We require sleep, food, and water to live. God is not limited. Our Creator does not slow down when He hasn't slept. He doesn't get dehydrated from lack of water.

If we only placed more trust in all of God's power, there would be no limits to what we could do. We could do more because we would have a supernatural power working on our behalf. We'd be calm and effective, gentle and kind—no matter how stressed.

Dear God, please be with me today. Every moment of my day, help me remember that I have You making the way, step by step. My ways, my view, and all I do is so limited. I know this and I am **STILL** quick to place my hope in only what I can see. Father, today I feel weary in doing good, doing right by others, especially if I feel they have not done right by me. Please God, help me remember that it is You Who takes care of me, You Who goes before me, and all I am asked to do is do good by others. You will indeed take care of the rest, so today help me trust You. I need to know and believe that all my days

I AM YOURS.

For the LORD God is our sun and our shield. He gives us grace
and glory. The LORD will withhold no good thing from those
who do what is right.

Psalm 84:11 NLT

LOVE MORE

God asked me to love more this morning. I asked Him, "How do
I do that?" He said,
Fear less, you are so protected.

We limit ourselves when we act from a place of fear, lack,
or not enough.

God's Spirit is readily available to anyone who asks.
Our Creator moves in mystical ways, and
He communicates love and support to
your heart.

God will whisper to you. It's low, soft, gentle, and
most of the time it's not what you are expecting,
but just what you need to hear.

Dear God, I know I need to be better at loving. I so easily meet my
friends and family with love, but people who hurt me? I oftentimes
fail at loving people I find hard to respect. Lord, whisper to me the
keys to love more. May my love be pure and a choice, may it be
true and honoring to You. God, it's in the gentle whisper where
I hear You. This Western world might name it intuition, but I call
it Your Holy Spirit. Your Spirit prompts an instinctive feeling deep
inside me that goes against my conscious reasoning! It appears in
the form of a gentle whisper or gut feeling, and it communicates
to me all I need. So please, keep whispering to me so I can
LOVE MORE.

After the wind there was an earthquake, but the LORD was not in the
earthquake. After the earthquake came a fire, but the LORD was not
in the fire. And after the fire came a gentle whisper.

1 Kings 19:11-12 NIV

I KNOW SHORTCUTS

Our Creator designed us, and He knows exactly what we need and when we need it. He wants nothing more than to give us what we need, but we simply forget to ask.

When I have an anxious mind, I do not think clearly. God knows shortcuts to your mind. He has the ability to open a door inside your brain and release all the useless thoughts that are flying around, causing you to stress.

God develops our spiritual instincts so we learn to turn to Him. His resourceful nature is greater than any difficulty we may ever face.

Dear God, please help me in my moments of distress. Show me Your door and open it, removing my stressful thoughts. God, help me to have peace as I walk through circumstances that feel larger than me and bless me with the courage to deliver. God, make a way that only You can make because, with You,
I KNOW SHORTCUTS.

Do not be anxious about anything, but in every situation, by prayer and petition, with thanksgiving, present your requests to God. And the peace of God, which transcends all understanding, will guard your hearts and your minds in Christ Jesus.

Philippians 4:6-7 NIV

REMEMBER WHO YOU ARE

You are my Creation
You are so loved, and
there is nothing I wouldn't do for you
Walk forward, move with this belief instilled in you

As you move throughout your day, give to others what you
would like to receive: compassion, a smile,
a compliment, the benefit of the doubt!

Life has a way of distracting you from what's important.
The more responsibility, the more excuses we give ourselves.

Lead with love today. May each person you meet feel rest
and a ray of light enter when they encounter you.

Dear Lord, I sometimes get so overwhelmed that I struggle to lead
with love. It's not that I am not kind, but I am not giving of my
time in the present moment because I am so stressed. It's not that
I am mean, but who is too busy for a smile? I know there must be
something wrong with this! Father, in times like these, I need You to
remind me who I am. I am Your divine creation, and I am loved, so
it is best that I freely love. Please help us do this on our slow days
and on our busy days so we can shift the atmosphere. Lord, when
I think of You, I love and work better. When I think of Your nature
and character, I lead better. Perhaps all I need to do is
REMEMBER WHO YOU ARE.

Be devoted to one another in love.
Honor one another above yourselves.

Romans 12:10 NIV

✦ MY PRESENCE ✦

One way our Creator shows His strength is by dwelling in and by people who are in challenging seasons of their lives. When the world 🌍 looks at their circumstances and says, "How do you still have a smile on your face?"

When God's hand is over your life, you increase in His likeness. God can make you feel light again, even if your load is heavy. He has the power to transcend your situation and bless you with joy.

Take your day moment by moment and simply:

Be present
Listen
Make eye contact
Love 💕

Dear God, there have been two seasons in my life when the pressing and squeezing were almost too much to bear, where I was forced to look to You daily for comfort and guidance. You showed up, and although each day was not overflowing with joy, I am happy to have made it through without giving up. Seeking You daily gave me strength. I pray more of Your children seek You to make it through so the world might look at them the way they looked at me and ask, "How could the smile be?" Oh, it's His presence that is within; it's God that is in
MY PRESENCE.

Seek the LORD and his strength; seek his presence continually!
1 Chronicles 16:11 ESV

DREAMS ARE FROM ME

I created more than just human life
There are angels that live in the heavenly realm with Me
And much more your minds cannot fathom
Know your precious life is close to Me
and I care to be present for every moment of it

We all have a purpose. We may not know our purpose
every day, but God does and He doesn't want you to
lose your fire 🔥 to ever dream a new dream.

Many of the things you do, I do, Vendy
I think, I have free will, I love, and part of Me is in you
I created you to dream because I dream, that's how
you came into existence

Dear Lord, I know dreams are from You because they take faith to
accomplish, and faith is of You. The greater the dream, the mightier
the faith it takes! Faith is what You speak of and desire Your children
to have. Dreams are real because You speak of them in the Old
Book, Your Scripture, the Holy Book! God, You created me after
a dream You had . . . You must have known I would choose You in
the face of many things. You must have thought of all the things that
would bring me to my knees, grow my heart, and protect me. You
must have placed in me a will to dream and a fire for You. You gave
me free will but also knew the test that would be placed in front of
me. So I ask You this, why me? Why did You choose me? What
dreams are from You, what purpose do You have for me aside from
dwelling close to You? Truthfully, there are days I question

everything, but coming back to You is the only thing that works for me. Will You fill my life with more prophecy so I know what dreams are from You and what

DREAMS ARE FROM ME?

And the Lord said, "Now hear what I have to say! When there are prophets among you, I reveal myself to them in visions and speak to them in dreams."

Numbers 12:6 GNT

MY TIMELINE IS DIVINE

Our Creator does not give us anything we cannot handle. We
are tested in many ways, but He sets us up for success, always.
Sometimes it's just a matter of sticking it out. And the very thing that
you were able to weather becomes your strength and roadmap.

No storm disturbs the soul that dwells close to
God, the Creator of all things.

Dear God, thank You for blessing me with sufferings.
I know nothing happens to me but for me, and asking for Your
guidance will make all the difference. Asking for Your peace. Asking
for Your perspective. Please, Lord, strengthen Your people all
around the world 🌍 and show them the way so they can experience
peace during our short and very temporary journey of life on earth.
🙏 Let us remember that it is You Who makes the way, You Who
gives peace that protects us, You Who guards our hearts
and minds. Father, with You
MY TIMELINE IS DIVINE.

And the peace of God, which transcends all understanding,
will guard your hearts and your minds in Christ Jesus.

Philippians 4:7 NIV

MY COURSE

Remember who you are
Remember all I brought you through
Remember to lead with love 🩶

God loves us so much. He holds us tight and doesn't want to let go. We may let go, we may forget, we may stray, but He never does.

By your Creator's side, you are protected. You may be attacked emotionally and spiritually, but God is stronger than anything you face.

Dear God, thank You for another day. Thank You for opening my eyes this morning. Thank You for Your love and encouragement. Help me to pass this along. Help me to be more like You. Help me choose Your path and stick to Your course. Thank You for Your protection today and to come. My God, I may be tested, but I pray to fight the good fight and stay by You. I know the mountains that form in my life will jump, leap, if I have You. Father, please help Your children stick to Your course, for only Your course is just and true. No longer will I choose *MY COURSE.*

"No weapon that is formed against you will succeed; And you will condemn every tongue that accuses you in judgment. This is the heritage of the servants of the LORD, And their vindication is from Me," declares the LORD.

Isaiah 54:17 NASB

I KNOW WHAT LIES AHEAD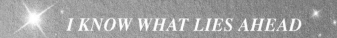

Our Creator made all things, and because He is not limited by time 🕐, He knows the exact course of your life. You choose every step of the way (it's part of having free will), but He already knows what You will decide because He is the beginning and the end.

Certain paths that seem impossible are placed there by God.

This should bring you comfort because you know the Creator of all things has a solution and a plan to get you through. He knows just how to get you through.

Ask for His guidance, and practice surrendering to Him.

Dear Lord, Your good and true purpose is my desire. I know You created the smith who blows fire in my coals. I know because the fire almost destroyed me, but since I chose You, I am now refined—a queen! In my kingdom, there is power and purpose for my daily regime, a weapon for Your kingdom. You have transformed me! My God, please continue to give Your people hope. When we doubt, give us signs placed at just the right time. Thanks to You, there are now many times where *I KNOW WHAT LIES AHEAD.*

See it is I who have created the smith who blows the fire
of coals, and produces a weapon fit for its purpose.

Isaiah 54:16 NRSV

MY THOUGHTS

Because our Creator is wiser and stronger than us, we will not fall. If your trust and confidence is in a power much greater than your own, and if you believe He is carrying you through your life, you know you will not be dropped. God could never—and would never—drop you. It's the safest place you could be, in His arms.

You may be in it, but your Creator is above it.

In His arms, you will find all your answers and the most perfect path.

Dear God, please help me to see, think, and move like You. Bless me with vision and thoughts ❀ that stem beyond my human understanding. Help me to see truth and spread light where I am at. 🐋 Father, Your ways are so much higher than my ways. Please give me a view from above so I can transcend all I am in. Please, I really need You. And as I wait, bless me with positive thoughts. Teach me to fight the bad ones off, for I want Your every thought and not
MY THOUGHTS.

"For my thoughts are not your thoughts, neither are your ways my ways," declares the Lord. "As the heavens are higher than the earth, so are my ways higher than your ways and my thoughts than your thoughts."

Isaiah 55:8-9 NIV

MY PEACE

Our Creator's peace transcends all understanding. It is gifted by
God, and only He can offer true peace in a broken world.

You are never alone. When you suffer, you are not
alone. There are people all around the world in
similar situations, with similar pains.

Ask for peace, and He will give it to you. Peace so
powerful, it can only come from God.

Dear Lord, I know this key is oh so true because I have experienced
it. You gave me peace when my heart was the most broken. When I
got home from work and cried myself to sleep day after day when
my father passed. I still have heavy days, but looking back on those
tear-filled mornings and evenings warms my heart. It warms my
heart because of how tenderly You held me. You held me when no
human could. No friend or family had the words or touch—it was
just You Who held my heart and spoke to my soul. It was just You
Who was there for me. I know there are many of Your children who
live far from You, who could never believe these words even if they
wanted to because I see now that it was a gift. My suffering was
truly a gift from You because the peace of mind and heart I have
will guard me no matter what hits. Fear no longer has a hold on me.
I walked through the valley of death and it sucked the life out of me
. . . It is meant to destroy and it almost did ruin me. But fear not,
troubled hearts, I promise this: He will give You peace.
Please just turn to Him, and look up!

There are three in one. My God, I hope my loss gives to Your
children who need it the most. Please share with them
my treasures and give them
MY PEACE.

I am leaving you with a gift—peace of mind and heart. And the peace
I give is a gift the world cannot give. So don't be troubled or afraid.

John 14:27 NLT

TRUST, LOVE, AND ENJOY

There are so many amazing memories I hold close to my heart.
I've been blessed with a beautiful life. However, this morning, as
I reflect, I realize the hardest times were some of the best times
because of how close I felt to God. I didn't think it was the best as
I was going through each one, but after, once all is said and done,
once you walk through the pain, you feel different.

My sweet Vendy, your life is moving so fast,
things change overnight
I need you to trust, love, and enjoy where your life is at
Because there is no such thing as ever going back

We can never go back.

Dear God, please help me to be present and enjoy my life with You.
With my family, friends, coworkers, and everyone You have put
in my path. Today will never come again. Open my eyes so I can
see my daily blessings and fill me with love, peace, and gratitude.
Remove my fear and stress. Show me what my human mind cannot
know without You. For today, I miss what was, and that's not the
direction You are taking me. I find, Lord, when it's just us, me and
You in my room, I am able to reset and be present for what's next.
Help me, Lord, fill me today, just enough to
TRUST, LOVE, AND ENJOY.

But when you pray, go away by yourself, shut the door behind
you, and pray to your Father in private. Then your Father, who
sees everything, will reward you.

Matthew 6:6 NLT

I AM HERE

We are not to worry. No matter how big or small your stress is, God doesn't want us to lose the peace He gives.

The word worry means "to be torn in two." That means your mind is one place and your body is another. Worry results in working against yourself.

The person Who spoke the most against worry had the biggest worry that ever existed. He came to this earth knowing He would be slaughtered and suffer more than any other person.

Our Creator has a living Spirit that is present all around the world 🌎 , and this Spirit can live inside you. It will guide you and give you answers you couldn't come up with on your own.

Dear Lord, I must thank You for Jesus. Your Son, in heaven He sat. At Your right hand He dwelt, and because of the will You placed on His heart, He journeyed down to earth. He knew what You sent Him to do would be hard, but He knew it would save each of us . . . So He left Your side and walked this earth. With two hands and two feet, He did many things: performed miracles that take faith to believe. What He did over two thousand years ago is not what draws me in . . . It's His ability to meet me where I am today in Playa del Rey, sitting on my bed, matcha in hand, with all my pain, knowing He carried the weight of the world and overcame. I must take heart, and I will because He made a way for His Spirit to dwell close to me. You see, this humble man Who has seen it all, says to me,

Sweet V, do not worry . . .
I AM HERE.

Do not worry about what to say or how to say it. At that time you will be given what to say, for it will not be you speaking, but the Spirit of your Father speaking through you.

Matthew 10:19-20 NIV

I PREPARE

Much of what God is doing in your life right now is preparing you. Preparing you for the next level. And if it weren't for your preparation, you would not be able to go—or even stay—where He would like to lead you next.

Trust that your Creator is making the way. Be grateful for today and the steps you have taken because there will be a time you look back and smile at it all. All that He was doing in your life.

Dear Lord, when a mother gives birth to her child, she intends to stay, keep her baby, and never walk away. She intends to watch her baby grow and learn how to do life. She knows for the first few months that her baby must remain close, glued to her breast to survive. The baby learns to thrive. That is where the baby takes in daily milk and sleeps best. The mother knows one day her child will grow and learn to do simple things, such as eat and drink, without her. She knows her baby will eventually know how to dress and shower on their own. She knows eventually her baby will grow to have children of their own, but even to old age, the mother will always care for the life she has brought into this world. My God, we live in a fallen, broken world where mothers have been separated from their babies at birth, and they do not get to experience watching them grow. Father, this is where Your mighty love moves in. The only thing stronger than the bond between a mother and her newborn baby is Your heart for us. Similar to how a mother endures labor pains and gives birth to a piece of her, You create us. We are part of You, and the great pain of the Son is what makes this oh so true.

God, I know You desire to feed me with Your milk and rock me
to sleep by Your side—that way I can grow. Grow to lead, think,
and reflect You in this world. You know I will make mistakes and
sometimes it is part of growing and learning. All I ask, Father, is that
I never live a life where I do not know You. You will always be my
Lord, my Father, and it's the natural, beautiful plans You have for me
that I would like to see. As I sit with You today, I know You are up
to mighty things in me. I can feel it in my bones, and as I learn to sit
with You more each day . . .

I PREPARE.

The LORD will work out his plans for my life—for your
faithful love, O LORD, endures forever. Don't abandon
me, for you made me.

Psalm 138:8 NLT

MY FEAR

Humility comes before honor.

If it weren't for the night that created a vulnerability in me,
how could I have compassion for all
I see that grows to honor me?
If it weren't for the way I humbly served,
how could I lead others who serve me?
If it weren't for the things that brought me to my knees,
what would have been noteworthy about what was accomplished
after all that broke me?
If it weren't for the wrong turns, mistakes, and pain in my eyes,
how could the decision to choose only
You be honoring?

The Creator of all things did not create you to fear
things of this world, or life itself, because He is in
control. The only thing to fear is His power.

Fear is an unpleasant feeling triggered by the perception of
danger—real or imagined. Fear is not given to us by God.
The only thing we are to fear is God Himself.

Nothing you face is greater than your Creator,
which means all things should fear Him.

Dear Lord, please remove every ounce of fear in my body and the
perceptions that live in my mind. Help me to see clearly. Help me to
live in a way where the only fear I have is of living a life that does
not honor You. My God, wisdom, she is so beautiful and she teaches
me. Her ways are much higher than mine, and she delights in truth.

I want to grow close to her because she instructs in ways that
honor You. As a result, her ways bring death to
MY FEAR.

Wisdom's instruction is to fear the LORD,
and humility comes before honor.

Proverbs 15:33 NIV

NOVEMBER

MY CLIMB

On our journey of life, we will have mountains—steep mountains—to climb. Ones where on your way up, rocks can and will fall. You may get scared and look back or look down!

Our Creator can take the mountain you are climbing and turn it on its side. The rocky edge now becomes the ground under you, and with Him, you are no longer scaling the side but crawling like a baby on top of the rocks.

Keep pushing, keep working, keep going! If you just keep going, He will begin to reveal more to you because only He knows just what you need to see or hear to make it through. His plans will begin to appear clearly, but you must keep climbing, chipping away, taking it day by day.

Dear Lord, sometimes Your climb seems too much for my little arms and feet. I am only 5'2" and there is much I cannot reach without You. Sometimes on my climb, it rains and pours. Sometimes the sun burns my back. Sometimes rocks fall, almost knocking me down This climb is **NOT** easy, but I guess that's the realization You would like Your children to come to . . . We were never designed to make it through without You. Our hearts, souls, and minds crave You. We crave the divine, something more . . . eternity! Things such as love, truth, and wisdom point to all of this. My God, as I grow tired on my climb, on the days life gets the best of me, please help me to not give up. I want to make it to the top of Your mountain. I can't wait to see the view that is from You. And on the days I grow weary of doing good, especially to others that bend a knee and serve You, please remind me that I was not designed to make it on my own. I was designed to scale the mountain with You. I will never be alone on *MY CLIMB.*

So let's not get tired of doing what is good. At just the right time we will reap a harvest of blessing if we don't give up.

Galatians 6:9 NLT

BE KIND AND PRESENT

Two very powerful things. One I'm great at, and the other,
I need some serious help with . . .

Kindness is the quality of being friendly, generous, and considerate.
Kindness is free; kindness is simple and the best thing you can
gift another human.

To be present in the moment takes work and practice. But it
has the power to further your relationships and
water your surroundings.

Wherever we are at, if we can just learn to
practice these two very simple things, our
lives will begin to flourish.

Dear Lord, there are seasons in my life where I just get so busy.
Sometimes, so much so that I lead with rushing, and kindness
takes a back seat. I am anxious and stressed, unable to see the
blessings because I am not present. My God, You speak of these
things—goodness, knowledge, self-control, perseverance, godliness,
affection, and love—so that in the midst of our crazy lives, no
matter what comes our way, we can always lead with
love. Oftentimes love means to
BE KIND AND PRESENT.

For this very reason, make every effort to add to your faith goodness; and to
goodness, knowledge; and to knowledge, self-control; and to self-control,
perseverance; and to perseverance, godliness; and to godliness, mutual
affection; and to mutual affection, love.

2 Peter 1:5-7 NIV

MY SPIRIT

That's the beauty of being in a relationship with Me,
I'm with you wherever you go
This means wherever you go in life,
you can bring joy with you
This means you are never alone
and nothing is too much for you to handle
You have Me, sweet V

Anything is possible with God. His ways will
surprise you and He never fails. Whatever you
need in this moment, in this stage of your life,
just invite His Spirit in. Ask His Spirit to guide you.
Ask in the moment, ask before bed, ask whenever
you get stressed, ask before you step into that big
meeting. All you have to do is ask.

And when He delivers, remember
Who provided for you.

Dear Lord, it is Your grace and Your Spirit that have been oh so
faithful to me. Not I, in comparison to You, I know nothing. You
have always provided for me when I turn to You. Your ways are so
good and true. You have even delivered me when I was not choosing
You. When my spirit was poor and my heart in two, You very
tenderly loved me. Because of this, I really want to give You my
best. I want You to have all of me. I want to choose You every day
and make up for the past times where I was stumbling

blind. Or the times I didn't choose You. I want to make up for my wrongs by living a life that honors and serves You. So please, protect my steps, continue to humble me, and let it be Your love that guides *MY SPIRIT.*

These are the ones I look on with favor: those
who are humble and contrite in spirit.

Isaiah 66:2 NIV

FROM ME

What if we actually believed every second of our lives that there is a higher power at work in our everyday life? Pushing you out of the way from getting hit by a car, whispering the answer in your ear when presenting to your boss, or gifting you with humility and understanding to say sorry to someone you love when you don't want to. All these little things add to your life and elevate your spirit. But oftentimes I think the weight of my life is all on me, and I find myself in a state of worry, which is like chasing after the wind.

Your Creator does exactly that. We may not always feel His presence, especially when we are stressed, but there is so much He does every moment for your daily protection.

Your Creator blesses you with understanding, wisdom, and answers when you need them most.

Your Creator protects. Nothing you accomplish is really just you.

Every win in my life comes from a divine hand that has led me there. I know this, and yet I forget and sometimes work as if it's all me, which leads to stress, fear, and depletion.

Dear God, today I ask for Your healing in all areas of my life. Help me to see that it's not me—it's You Who takes care. Help me to enjoy each day and see all the beauty and good You have created and placed before me. A dream of mine, and maybe Yours as well, is to see more of Your creation, more of Your children, walk in freedom. Freedom from shame, freedom from fear. Freedom from all that robs them of their peace. Father, I know this dream of mine comes from the many cares You have placed on my heart. Cares for the poor in spirit, women, children, orphans, the fatherless, and the mentally distressed! Lord, please deliver us from the evil that rules in this world. Equip Your children, strengthen them in Your words, grow them in Your wisdom, and empower them to fight the battle that takes place but is unseen. Father, continue to write cares on my heart and plant new dreams, for it is all You moving in me and never *FROM ME.*

A dream comes when there are many cares.

Ecclesiastes 5:3 NIV

✦ TIME WITH ME ✦

You grow in fullness the more time you spend with Me
I pour into you, your spirit is calm, you radiate light
And you are able to give more
of what little time and energy you have
Because it's all Me

The more time you spend with your Creator, the more
trust is built because you start to see the power of
His Spirit move in your everyday life.

Trust in my Creator gives me confidence. The more I can trust in
God's plan for my life, the more peace I have. The better
I perform.

Trust in my Creator provides reliability when I'm lost, truth when
I'm confused, ability when I'm discouraged, and strength
when I'm weak.

Dear God, I do love my time with You. Most days, especially on the
days it takes much effort to be still and protect time with You, You
give me just the right keys to unlock what I need. The more time we
spend together, the more my faith grows because I get to see Your
character, which is so true. It allows me to rest and trust in this truth.
I know You would never lie to me, You would never leave me, You
would never be unkind to me, You would never not love me.
I wish more people, but especially women, had more time with
You because it would plant so much good in the world.

I wish more men spent more time with You because it would create mighty change. My God, thank You for the perfect peace You have given me. May my heart, eyes, and mind always seek You first so others may be encouraged after spending
TIME WITH ME.

You will keep him in perfect peace, whose mind
is stayed on You, because he trusts in You.

Isaiah 26:3 MEV

YOU ARE NOT ALONE

We have a team. Our Creator blesses us with
helping hands, loving family, friends, and
people full of compassion as we journey
through life.

At times I tend to push away these helping hands. I'm so fearful
of being a burden that I fail to communicate, I fail to love, I fail
to find comfort in the help that God sends my way. Then I feel
overwhelmed and shut down.

Dear God, please guide me today. Help me to use my team and
resources that bring light, love, and joy to my life. I ask for a grateful
and joy-filled heart. 🤍 After all, I am only twenty-four years old
with no children of my own and no life to take care of but my own!
I ask for guidance and help in the areas where I need more support
because today will simply never come again and to isolate myself
due to my shortcomings at such a young and tender age does no
good. My God, I pray for Your youth, may they look to the sunny
sky and smile, take in the breeze and giggle until it hurts. May they
scream for ice cream, jump for joy on half days and free dress (😖
it's the Catholic schoolgirl in me), and know that all things will
happen in due time. May they know there is a loving Creator in
charge, and no matter what happens in life, they are never alone.
Lord, with You none of us are ever alone. Please speak to the souls
who need to hear this most, whisper to the depths of their hearts,
YOU ARE NOT ALONE.

You who are young, be happy while you are young, and
let your heart give you joy in the days of your youth.

Ecclesiastes 11:9 NIV

✦ IN ME ✦

Uncertainty, change, failure, growth
Through all the variables of life,
I am the only One that can grant
you true happiness and peace
Invite Me in, talk to Me throughout your day,
smile up at Me, thank Me,
I'm here to comfort you
I'm the only thing that can grant you certainty
and stability in an unstable world

Your job, relationships, home, and passions could all change or be gone tomorrow. Nothing this world 🌎 offers is forever. There are few things that feed your soul, but they are what matter most.

God is truly the only reliable factor in your life. Unlike human relationships, the safest thing to do is place all of your expectations and trust in this relationship, which then causes you to become more full.

I have not believed this my entire life, nor do I always do this. I've lived a very blessed life, full of love, support, and comfort, but when all the things I placed so much of my trust in fell apart, the only thing holding me together was God's love.

Family, friends, lovers, and dreams are all wonderful, but none of those things offer true consistency. They could all be gone tomorrow. Of course, be thankful for all the beauty you've been blessed with and enjoy it while it's yours, but know that these things can and will never be enough.

Bruised hearts I heal
Hope I restore
Life I give
Fullness
You will
Only find in Me

Dear Lord, there is so much You speak to me. Much of what You say will come to pass, but in the moment it all surpasses my knowledge. It even surpasses my beliefs. You tell me these things because I spend much time with You. I am still learning how to navigate the pain that lives in my eyes, and at times I feel it has hardened me. But the more I choose You, the more filled with Your Spirit I am, which in return softens me. You delight in my strength and ability to choose You, but hardness is not what You desire for me. To be hard in a hard and cold world is to be hardened by the hard and cold world. Full of compassion and mercy, tenderhearted, is the design You desire for us all, but it takes much time with You for healing and restoration to take place
IN ME.

And to know the love of Christ that surpasses knowledge,
that you may be filled with all the fullness of God.

Ephesians 3:19 ESV

✦ MY PROMISE ✦

My words are truth because I am God
My words have power because I am God
My words are living because I am God

God = The Creator and ruler of the universe and source of
all moral authority; the supreme being.

When a human makes a promise, there is a chance it will be
broken. When your Creator makes a promise, it's already done.

Take comfort today knowing that God is in control
and His promise to love and take care of you is
unmatched compared to the flawed nature of humanity.
If your Creator made a promise to you, it's already
done. Live in that space with hope and peace for
all that is to come.

Dear Lord, every morning You are my strength. I have learned to
turn to You. Now, I turn to You whether it's sunny or rainy. And
because I turn to You with my mornings, I have learned that it is
there in the stillness I hear from You. Because I now hear from
You, I know Your promises. Your mighty plans and beautiful
promises for my life fuel me and comfort me. Lord, I pray for more
of Your children to wake each morning and learn of Your promises
for their lives. My God, I pray to always belong to You. May
Your heart bring delight to
MY PROMISE.

LORD, be gracious to us; we long for you;
and be our strength every morning.

Isaiah 33:2 ISV

YOU ARE CHOSEN

You are chosen to love. You are chosen to serve. You are chosen
to play. You are chosen to work. You are chosen to be a friend.
You are chosen to be a wife or husband.

We have callings in our lives—roles we get to play.
Some are seasonal, some are permanent. Our
Creator has the power to fill in the gaps so that
whenever we fall short, He steps in.

Dear God, thank You for choosing me. Thank You for guiding me.
I ask that as You continue to choose me and people all over the
world 🌍 , You strengthen us in Your love so we can walk with
humility and light. So we can do right by You and others. God, I
pray for people who are being challenged, people whom You are
growing in this season of their lives. I ask that You give them the
courage they need to keep going. May their perseverance result in
a blessing much greater than they could have imagined. May they
know it was by Your hands and Your hands only . . . they are chosen.
Now I consider it pure joy to know the trials, the many sufferings
I have faced in my short time on earth, have served as a training
for the divine. A training for a massive outpouring of Your Spirit.
Perseverance will finish its work in me because You have appointed
me, and by the blood of Jesus, I can do the impossible. When I was
on my knees, it was You Who said to me,

Get up! Vendela,
YOU ARE CHOSEN.

Consider it pure joy, my brothers and sisters, whenever you face trials of many
kinds, because you know that the testing of your faith produces perseverance.
Let perseverance finish its work so that you may be mature and complete,
not lacking anything.

James 1:2-4 NIV

MY HEART

Let Me bless you
You are My child and
I want to gift you with a beautiful life
One filled with joy, excitement, love, passion,
and deep purpose
One filled with hope and honor
One filled with the fruits of My Spirit

God wants to see you and all your loved ones thrive. He wants to see us live abundant lives, filled with His peace.

Our Creator receives so much joy when we flourish. Your Creator wants to see your life flourish in all areas, not just one. The good news is He has the power to do this. To transform every area of your life and use everything for your good.

Dear God, today I put every moment in Your hands. I thank You for all Your love. Help me to enjoy the many daily blessings and open my eyes to them. God, I thank You for Your unmeasurable goodness. I pray for Your will in the lives of all people because what You have planned is far greater than anything the human mind could come up with. Father, this world is not used to a love like Yours. It is foreign and so pure. Compassion that pours out and warms my body like a blanket during a windy sunset at the beach, and faithfulness so true it pumps blood to
MY HEART.

The Lord, the Lord, the compassionate and gracious God,
slow to anger, abounding in love and faithfulness.

Exodus 34:6 NIV

NO MEASURE

There is no measure to what I can do
Even now

There is nothing our Creator cannot do. Everything in your life can serve a greater purpose.

God had used difficult situations in my life so I could learn to trust Him completely. My life and surroundings are determined by God, Who knows what is best for me, and I am learning to bend a knee to whatever God gives.

God takes us through different levels of life; how we handle each stage will determine how long we are there. My life has been filled with many waiting seasons, and the minute I surrender and truly bend a knee to Him is usually when He opens the door to my next chapter.

God's timeline is divine. Allow Him to continue to grow you where you are because He is preparing you for all that is next.

If it weren't for the training now, you couldn't possibly handle what's next.

Dear Lord, I write to You today from a coffee shop, and I am truly excited for all that is next. Reflecting on my writings, many prayers, and journaling, I see how You have tested me. I see how You have grown me. I see how heavy my heart was and tears come to my eyes because I was such a light, but for so long my light went out.

For what felt like so long, I was down. A wet blanket covered my life, but You spoke to me during these times and told me of the many promises that are to come. I pray we look forward and up, letting go of the past. I pray we learn to praise You more. There is truly no such thing as understanding Your greatness, but praising You will help us make it through—for there is no limit to what You can do, absolutely NO MEASURE.

The LORD is great and is to be highly praised; his greatness
is beyond understanding.

Psalm 145:3 GNT

✦ *ALL THINGS* ✦

No amount of pain, suffering, injustice, or fear is too
great for God.

He's seen it all because He created it all. Whatever you have gone
through doesn't worry Him; what worries Him is when you try to do
things on your own, for you were designed to rest in
your Creator.

It's easy for me to think God is overwhelmed when I am
overwhelmed. It's easy for me to see limits because I'm
a limited human.

One year ago today, I lost my dad. I'm now learning how to hand
things over to my Creator, Who carries it all. It was too much for me
and my best choice was to look to Him.

There is nothing He can't do, especially with your pain.
He loves using your pain to transform you. 🤍

Wherever you are on this journey, know that what feels
too hard or heavy for you probably is. The Creator of
the universe can do a much better job with it than you
can, so invite Him in.

Dear God, the Creator of all things, is anything too hard for
You? Are You not in charge, can You not command
ALL THINGS?

I am the LORD, the God of all mankind. Is anything too hard for me?

Jeremiah 32:27 NIV

FOUNDATION IN ME

Vendy, I have to bring you through certain things
So you know your foundation,
So you know what you can truly rely on in this world
So you can learn to choose Me

To rely is to depend on with full trust or confidence.

With His love, you can accomplish what would
otherwise be impossible on your own.

Dear Lord, I am struggling because I keep asking, **WHY?** I keep
asking myself, **WHY** do You let certain things happen? **WHY** must
breaking be part of the process, part of the journey? I want to be
restored to my bliss-filled, carefree self. Naivety . . . sure, but some
days I wish to go back. Hardened I never was, but this is what truly
hurts me. Needing, wanting to know the **WHY** is not of Your design.
You simply want me to trust You Who is able to do immeasurably
more than all I ask or see, than all I imagine, as long as it is
according to Your will for me. Father, please remove my desire to
know the **WHY**. For, in time, You reveal all things to me I need.
Keep me focused on You, for that is the best
FOUNDATION IN ME.

Now to him who is able to do immeasurably more than
all we ask or imagine, according to his power that is at
work within us.

Ephesians 3:20 NIV

NEW GROUND

Vendy, it's not going to stop, it's just the beginning
Transformation is happening
It is taking place and I am moving in the hearts of
My people everywhere
I give My people a new lens, and with this comes strength
to do what's right
And drive for their future

God completes the will He has for you. All
you must do is trust Him with each step.

Dear God, today I pray to love more. I pray You would grow my
knowledge and depth of insight so I can discern what is best and
pure for myself and others. You have started a mighty work in me,
the training has taken place since I was a little girl, but it picked up
major speed when You took him, AJ, from me. Since then, You have
blessed me with a new lens and a hunger for only Your will. I have
transformed into something new, something sculpted by You. I am
confident that what You are doing in me is something oh so mighty,
and I can let go of all that is next because You will carry it all out.
I can't wait to see the sprouted seeds in my soil and the beautiful
terrain, oh the territory and
NEW GROUND.

Being confident of this, that he who began a good work
in you will carry it on to completion until the day of
Christ Jesus.

Philippians 1:6 NIV

HEALING

One of My greatest gifts 📖 is healing
I bless souls who come to Me with restoration
and hope in all areas
Healing comes through love,
and it takes many different forms
I have the power to restore everything and anything

Our Creator heals our minds, bodies, and souls.
There is nothing He cannot heal.

God, I am grateful for the healing You have blessed me with this past year. It's so powerful; I hope others receive Your healing in whatever area of life they need.

My healing is more vast than the ocean 🌊
I have never-ending streams of it
Just ask Me now what area you need it most and
I will send a wave

Dear Father, much healing and restoration needed to take place in me. Trauma I didn't even know I had, pains I didn't know existed, and a lifetime of moving at a speed that did not feed me. My Lord, You are oh so good and the healing You offer is not of this world. It transcends. Reading my past journal entries, I can see that it was always You Who brought balm to my wounds. You have restored me to health. Healing is the most therapeutic thing because we live on earth and dwell in a land that is far from You. We all need much of Your healing. And if we do not take the time to heal, Father, we move at a speed that brings mighty hurt to others. Please keep the healing flowing with every wave in the sea, and bring this beautiful thing to all Your creation because it's our minds, bodies, and souls that crave and need Your

HEALING.

"But I will restore you to health and heal your wounds," declares the LORD.

Jeremiah 30:17 NIV

DECEMBER

ASHAMED OF YOUR PAIN

When I think of the life of my Savior . . . If I were to look directly into His eyes, I'd see life, hope, and the pain of this world.

You know what you've weathered and how much you can truly handle. I can easily think of the pain I've experienced through loss as setting me back in my life, or I can choose to see it as something that launched me forward. I have felt extremely insecure about my pain, wanting to pretend it's not there, but that does nothing for me or others.

Don't be ashamed of your pain. It has the power to grow you, bring comfort to others, and make you stronger.

The greatest people in history who have changed the world endured pain of unfathomable levels. My God endured pain more than any other human.

Now, when you look into my eyes 👀 , you may see pain that was never there before, but God has the power to heal our pain and tenderize our hearts. 🤍 Never feel ashamed of your pain because it can actually be the greatest advantage you have. It can be the one thing that sets you apart, propels you forward, and changes the world!

Dear Lord, thank You for the pain! It's not that I want more of it or desire it, but I welcome it because, when I am afflicted, I learn of Your authority. We may welcome it, but it's okay for us to never love it, but rather love what it does to our flesh. It makes it so the Spirit in us rises in power and authority, rather than the flesh ruling our steps! Oh, how it was good for me to be afflicted; I have learned to take the pain and create. I write my pain, I watch the sunset with my pain, I go for long walks with my pain, I drink lots of hot tea with my pain, I use my pain to pray, and I even help others with my pain! So, children of God, may He strengthen you and empower you so you are never again

ASHAMED OF YOUR PAIN.

It was good for me to be afflicted so
that I might learn your decrees.

Psalm 119:71 NIV

FAITH FOR TODAY

You don't know what is around the corner, but I do
You don't know what each day holds, but I do
Therefore, all I ask is that you
have enough faith for Me each day

Seconds lead to minutes, which result in hours. Then
hours turn into a full day, and that day leads to
365 days, which make up a year. The years grow and
grow, turning into a lifetime of faith . . . but all you
need is enough to get you through today!

What I am doing does not always make sense
in the moment, which is why you need faith
I have a way of building you, expanding your mind,
growing your heart
And strengthening your ability to recognize
Me throughout your each day

Dear God, please grant me enough faith for today so I can be
grateful and joyful for all You have blessed me with. So I can put
my best foot forward, knowing it is You guiding each step. When
I have faith for the day, it multiplies and results in me becoming a
faithful person who You so beautifully bless! Please show us
what it means and looks like to have enough
FAITH FOR TODAY.

A faithful person will be richly blessed.

Proverbs 28:20 NIRV

DAYS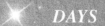

There will be good days and bad days. If you never had a bad
day, then you wouldn't know what a good day felt like!

You will have dry seasons, seasons of waiting, and fulfilling
seasons. All seasons are part of life. All seasons will come and
all seasons will pass.

There is nothing God cannot restore or give strength
to. Fight to keep your spirits up and look ahead,
knowing the beautiful sun will rise again
to present a new day.

Dear God, You promise to never cause pain without allowing
something new to be born. To clarify, You are not the author of pain,
but You are the most powerful force, which means You allow pain
to happen. You allow the pain to happen due to free will. Of course,
Your desire for us is to choose You, but it could never be a choice
unless we had free will. Therefore, pain is a byproduct and not what
You intended for the world, but You are so good that pain becomes
a solution if we choose to hand it over to You! Father, on my good
days and on my bad days, for all my days, please remind me that
the pain I see is the byproduct of a fallen world, and You allow us
to walk through it only to use it for our good, to create something
new for all our
DAYS!

"I will not cause pain without allowing something
new to be born," says the LORD.

Isaiah 66:9 NCV

ENJOY THE RIDE

It's not always easy to keep a healthy perspective in a life that is filled with so many twists and turns. A healthy outlook on life takes practice. You have to mentally put boundaries up and learn to train your mind so when thoughts come in that do not benefit you, you are able to make a U-turn and drive in a different direction.

Your attitude, your point of view, determines whether you enjoy your life or don't enjoy your life.

Since I was a little girl, I've always loved wisdom: the quality of having experience, knowledge, and good judgment. I have not always made wise decisions, but I've always been hungry for a deeper understanding. I have always had a hunger for wisdom.

God created wisdom before He created this earth—before He created you and me.

The LORD brought me forth as
the first of His works.

Proverbs 8:22 NIV

Dear God, please grant me wisdom on this journey of life. Her fruits are beautiful, and it is wisdom, her guidance, that broadens my perspective so I can
ENJOY THE RIDE.

I love those who love me, and those
who seek me find me.

Proverbs 8:17 NIV

HURT

People will hurt you. You will do things that hurt you. Hurt is a powerful emotion. It can ruin friendships, marriages . . . pretty much any type of relationship.

When we hold on to hurt, it hardens our hearts ♡ and ruins our relationships because we replace love with hurt.

This morning, God asked that I give my hurt to Him. I had a vision where I handed my hurt over to God and it was wrapped in a little red box with a bow. He said He would take care of it.

When people hurt you, you must forgive. When you hurt yourself, you must forgive. Part of forgiveness is surrendering the hurt to God and trusting that He will take good care of this box. He will free you so you are lighter. God does not remove the hurt, but He will bring restoration and peace.

The hurtful action or thing that requires forgiveness may never go away, but your ability to forgive makes it so it doesn't have to.

When you hand your box of hurt over to God, He simply says,

I'll take care of it. Now let me bring you comfort and please communicate love to that person. Continue to love yourself. I got this.

Dear God, there is much about forgiveness You would like to teach me. First, forgiveness is more for our own benefit than anything else. Second, if I do not learn to forgive, and forgive more quickly, I will postpone the healing and the glorious plans You have for me. Third, the more I practice forgivingness, the happier I am because it will be part of every stage of my life. We will always be called to forgive, and as long as we are doing life with others, there will be plenty of opportunities to exercise forgiveness. God, You have blessed me with so much love in my life. I have amazing friends, the most loving and supportive family, but the minute I come across someone who hurts me, I am quick to build a wall and try to protect myself. I also find I more easily forgive someone I love, but I am less likely to forgive someone I do not love. Father, I pray for more love to fill my heart and people's hearts everywhere—that way we can walk in true freedom, which is birthed from forgiveness. Father, I grow in wisdom the more I hand my box of hurts over to You and forgive. For I know it is the desire of Your heart for us to release all our *HURT*.

A person's wisdom yields patience; it is to one's
glory to overlook an offense.

Proverbs 19:11 NIV

PAINT THE STARS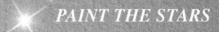

There are about one hundred thousand million stars in the Milky Way and God placed each individual star ⭐ in the sky.

God wants us to paint 🌠 the sky with Him.

Vendy, I'm with you
I'm your God and I'm the only One
that has the power to paint the sky
I'm the only One that has the
power to take your hand and paint the sky
I'm with you and I'm showing you with
my divine hand how to paint the sky
I want you to enjoy what I'm doing
Relax and be in awe because you're doing
what is impossible to do on your own
I'm holding your hand tight

Ask God's Spirit for more of Its guiding grace, and pray for less of your limited ways.

You. Your carefree, childlike self is who God wants to paint and create with. It's easy and magical with Him.

Dear Lord, I don't have the power to paint the sky, but when I take Your hand and together we poke at the sky, suddenly I am painting stars ⭐ in the universe. This means I can do the impossible with

You holding my hand. Whatever is Your true and good will for me and my life, may Your purpose be painted in the sky and reflected in my life. Please, together let's
PAINT THE STARS.

For it is God who works in you to will and
to act in order to fulfill his good purpose.

Philippians 2:13 NIV

CONFIDENCE

Confidence is the feeling or belief that one can rely on someone or something; it means to have a firm trust in someone.

When we find confidence in things that are fleeting, we become weak because the ground we are standing on starts to crack. When your world falls apart, but the ground you're standing on is firm, you are able to stand strong.

God, help me to place more trust in Who You are and all You do. Help me because I so often forget. Help me so I can move forward with peace.

Dear God, I ask that my confidence be in You. When this happens, I forgive better, my relationships are better, I perform better, I love better, and my life is more full. Please, God, bless me with Your humility, grace, and
CONFIDENCE.

But blessed is the one who trusts in the
LORD, whose confidence is in him.

Jeremiah 17:7 NIV

FOREVER JOURNEY

Doing what is honorable is for our own freedom. To be free of unhealthy emotions is a constant process based on the choices we make. When we choose truth, kindness, and honesty, and act from that place, we become blameless.

When I choose to eat an apple 🍎 over candy 🍬 , even if candy is what I want in the moment, I know it's a small win for my health. I know I will not always choose the apple, but humility and love bring me back to center.

True: In accordance with facts or realities.

Noble: Having or showing good personal qualities.

Right: Morally justified, or acceptable.

Pure: Free of contamination.

Lovely: Exquisitely beautiful, pleasing.

Admirable: Arousing or deserving respect, honor.

Humble yourself and lead with love, and there you will find more joy in your everyday life.

Dear Father, today I pray more of Your children learn to choose the apple over the candy! Candy is yummy and has its place in life, but the apple feeds our bodies and offers nutrients that fuel us. When we make decisions that are honoring to our bodies and minds, we walk in freedom. Meditating on all that is noble, right, pure, lovely, and admirable is a lifelong skill and something to cultivate. When we focus on all that is praiseworthy, we feed our minds, so we are more likely to choose the apple on our *FOREVER JOURNEY.*

Finally, brothers and sisters, whatever is true, whatever is noble, whatever is right, whatever is pure, whatever is lovely, whatever is admirable—if anything is excellent or praiseworthy—think about such things.

Philippians 4:8 NIV

MY FAITHFUL LOVE

Looking back, both the most challenging moments and the best moments in my life all came from God.

The pain-filled moments He used to grow me, deepen my understanding, and expand my vision. The joy-filled moments usually surrounded me with love. Loving God, myself, and others pushed me forward and helped me accomplish whatever I put my mind to.

The good days, God is there. The bad days, He is there. We are never truly alone, and because of this the night will never hold you down.

Dear God, thank You for loving me so much. For speaking life into me and for guiding me. I pray You do the same for others, and I pray for more people to hear from You and draw near to You. Your love is so powerful, Your comfort is so great, and You have a never-ending supply of wisdom, love, courage, and strength. I know that in whatever lies ahead, I will always have You, *MY FAITHFUL LOVE.* 🤍

And so we know and rely on the love God has for us. God is love. Whoever lives in love lives in God and God in them.

1 John 4:16 NIV

NOTHING I WOULDN'T DO FOR YOU

The closer I get to you, the more full you feel
When I consume your mind and heart,
nothing will harm you
There are powers and forces working every day
that you have zero control over
It's important to know this, but not to focus on this
Vendy, My Spirit is enough
What I have left you with on earth will be enough
I perform miracles with a single word
You strive a lifetime for what I can bless you with in a moment,
through a single word
So turn to me for your every desire
There is nothing I wouldn't do for you

You must believe there is nothing God wouldn't
do for you. You must know there is nothing
too great for God.

Dear God, thank You for all You have done for me. I will never be
able to thank You enough, nor will I ever understand all You have
done for me because much of the work You do on my behalf I don't
even see! And because I cannot see so much of it, I fall into the
trap of thinking anything I accomplish is my doing. Oh, foolish me!
My God, it is You, it has always been You. Your Spirit guiding me,

teaching me what to say and how to say it. So the next time I stress for what is next, please remind my heart and mind in the gentle ways You do. I love You, God. Create in me a faithful soul, for there is *NOTHING I WOULDN'T DO FOR YOU.*

Do not worry about what to say or how to say it. At that time you will be given what to say, for it will not be you speaking, but the Spirit of your Father speaking through you.

Matthew 10:19-20 NIV

RECOGNIZED BY FRUIT

I'd like to be recognized as a hardworking and caring person. Generous in spirit and giving. Compassionate and strong. Humble yet confident.

How do you recognize qualities in a person? It's their actions that form a reputation. Daily acts begin to define them due to the consistency of these acts.

How do you want to be recognized? What does it look like to be recognized as this?

Dear God, help me be recognized due to Your Spirit that lives in me. Something that is different, supernatural, and not of this world! May this world recognize me and see You because they recognize the fruits that are from You! May more of Your children produce fruit and be
RECOGNIZED BY FRUIT.

Make a tree good and its fruit will be good, or make a tree bad
and its fruit will be bad, for a tree is recognized by its fruit.

Matthew 12:33 NIV

SOLITARY WITH ME

Some of my most fond memories have been when I'm alone.
Listening to music 🎵 while cooking at sunset with the ocean breeze
flowing into my home.

When my dad passed, that's what I needed most. I needed time alone
to heal, process, cry, and talk to God. I needed time alone because
that's when I hear from my Creator best. I am now in a place where I
don't need as much alone time, but I enjoy it and crave it, which is a
blessing that stems from the pain.

Peace with being alone has been one of the greatest
gifts to my life. I've learned so much about myself,
and I've grown in my confidence.

Suffering soul
Take heart
During your
Solitary time with Him
He will teach you
To meet with truth the lies
That fill your mind
Suffering soul
Continue to do as He did
As He instructs
And withdraw to your
Solitary time

The more I learn about the life of Jesus, the more patterns
I pick up on. He would retreat from the world 🌍 to be with His
Father. If the most powerful human that ever walked the land
did this to recharge, imagine what it could do for your life . . .

Dear Lord, I pray for more time with You. Even though my heart is not breaking the way it did before, I always want to crave this time because it sets me free. It frees me from the lies in my mind! Please always protect and keep *SOLITARY WITH ME*.

When Jesus heard what had happened, he withdrew
by boat privately to a solitary place.

Matthew 14:13 NIV

MY DAYS

When you don't stop to smell the roses 🌹, much of the beauty
in life passes you by. Over and over again.

Vendy, please enjoy today
It's a gift from Me

You are allowed to enjoy every moment of your
life, especially because some moments will be
more challenging to enjoy than others.

On the days you can rest,
rest and allow me to restore you
On the days you can celebrate, celebrate
On the days you need to work, go for it

Sometimes desires get in the way. That longing for what you don't
have has the ability to rob you of what's in front of you. It makes the
journey of life seem so drawn out.

I created you to have certain desires
I placed them in your heart and the more you trust
and get to know Me
The more you realize how much I care
to see them fulfilled
The more you know the outcome is in my hands
The safest place it could be
If you knew how much I loved you,

you would enjoy your life more
With Me it is all already done
You would take in each stage you are in
and savor it because it will not come again

God keeps us moving forward, and if we saw
His every move, we would be filled with
gratitude because of all the new
things He continues to do.

Dear Lord, You continue to extend Your hand to me. Me of
teeny-tiny faith, You are constantly extending Your hand to me!
Because of this, I am able to see each day as a gift. I know all I have
to do is turn to You when I grow distressed. Take the burning desires
You placed on each of our hearts and hold them in Your hand, the
safest place they could be. Keep them warm until I am ready, free
from doubt, and then take my hand and promise to be with me all
MY DAYS.

Immediately Jesus reached out his hand and caught him.
"You of little faith," he said, "why did you doubt?"

Matthew 14:31 NIV

DIVINE PLAN

I just need you to trust, My sweet daughter
I don't waste time.
With Me everything is strung together
in the best way possible
Trust Me and I will make it clear.
I will direct you like I have in the past
Continue to check in with Me,
never letting worry overcome you
I move and make things happen on My divine timeline
There is not much for you to do but trust Me

While you are on this journey, continue to keep His ways.
You may not have the answer at every turn, but with
God, answers are not what you need. It is His wisdom
that will protect your ways and guide your every step.

Dear Lord, I know You have a very special plan for my life. I know
this because You would whisper to my heart when I was a little girl,
and as I grew and walked through things that hurt me, You kept
reminding me of the beautiful life You were creating for me, if I
could just keep the faith, hold on tight to You, and fight the good
fight! Do what I know is right and true in my heart and simply bend
a knee to You. I am starting to see the pieces fall into place. I know
these writings are a sign that point to Your divine timeline. But,
Father, what I must do is pray to remain humble and close to You,
no matter the new heights You take me to, or how often the view
changes, I must remain faithful to You. And remaining faithful to
You is reflected in how I treat others,

Your sheep! Father, I pray for kindness all around. I pray to move, act, serve, and live in kindness. This does not mean I lead with fake smiles or charm that deceives, but rather give and expect nothing in return, forgive freely, and let this generosity pave the way because it all points to You and Your

DIVINE PLAN.

Give, and it will be given to you. A good measure, pressed down, shaken together and running over, will be poured into your lap. For with the measure you use, it will be measured to you.

Luke 6:38 NIV

AFRAID TO LOVE

Vendy, you hold back the love you feel
because you are afraid to get hurt
You hold back because you are
afraid to be seen and
you think it may not be enough

You will get hurt—that's part of love. When you love someone or something, they have the power to hurt you. They have the power to hurt themselves, which in turn can also hurt you! Yes, it's easier not to care, easier not to love, but you lose out on so much.

Don't be afraid to love. The biggest lie is thinking you are protecting yourself by not loving.

Show your heart. It's okay to have an open heart in all areas of your life. The world needs more of you and more of your heart.

The largest hurt in my life stems from not loving fully.

Dear Lord, boy have You taught me a lot about love these past few years. I never once feared my father because our love was so pure. He made me feel as if there was nothing I could ever do for him to love me less. Our love was perfect. We were not perfect. My father was not perfect and I am not perfect, but I know for a fact that our love was. It was the strongest love I have ever received from a man. Which is why it hurts me so much now to love. I am tempted to hold back and I am filled with fear, especially when it comes to dating.

Not because I fear a broken heart. I have already experienced the loss of love when my father passed. But mighty fear in facing the consequences that stem from a broken heart. The way we start to compare ourselves and look in the mirror as if there is something wrong with us, as if we are not enough due to the lack of love. Well, Your love is the only thing that has cast away any fear I might have. Fear of being not enough or too much. Fear fear fear that has stopped me from doing all You have placed on my heart to do! So I thank You, Father, for casting away the fears that make us

AFRAID TO LOVE.

There is no fear in love. But perfect love drives out fear, because fear has to do with punishment. The one who fears is not made perfect in love.

1 John 4:18 NIV

BOUNDARIES TO LOVE

When I don't get enough rest, I break out in cold sores. When my body is stressed, my immune system picks it up. It's my body's way of telling me to recharge. Large, juicy cold sores grow on my lips and itch.

My soul, similar to my body, has needs. I can feed the flesh with rest, water, and sleep to avoid cold sores. But how do I feed my soul?

I feel my heart 🩶 growing a cold sore when I don't experience enough alone time with God. My mind is weak and I'm run down because I'm not doing the one thing that feeds me the most. I am not resting with my Creator Who casts away lies with His truth. He fights off my soul's cold sores.

Doing more can result in less. The key is to do more of what feeds you.

Vendy, do I put boundaries on My love for you?
The more you allow Me in, the more I can lead the way

God grants you the ability to love more fully. To love someone with all their shortcomings. To love yourself with all your shortcomings. He takes away our cold sores with His everlasting love.

Do as He does: Place no limits on Your love and turn to Him for more. His is consistent and unfailing.

Dear Lord, teach me to love like You. I want to remove the boundaries on the love You place in my life and on my heart; I want this love to be full and everlasting like You. Keep me faithful to You, Father; keep me faithful to Your love, and remove my *BOUNDARIES TO LOVE*.

The LORD appeared to him from far away. I have loved you with an everlasting love; therefore I have continued my faithfulness to you.

Jeremiah 31:3 ESV

JANUARY

✦ *GREATEST COMMAND* ✦

When the Pharisees asked Jesus what the greatest law was,
He replied *love*. Love God, and secondly, love your
neighbor as yourself.

So much to unpack with love. It's not easy to love God and put Him
first, and it's definitely not easy to love people in the same way you
love yourself or your family and friends.

God, what can I do to better uphold these truths?

More of Me, sweet V, is all you need

More time with God = more of His Holy Spirit,
which lives in each of us and guides us while
we are in human form here on earth. His Spirit
will teach you how to love.

I notice when I don't have my alone time with God, the color in my
life is not as vibrant and I struggle to love in full capacity.

God's most important command is to **LOVE**.

If we can all practice loving a bit more today, we'd be putting a
smile on the face that created all things. That's powerful.

Dear Lord, Jesus said the most important of Your commands is to
love. He was a very special man, and it is His love that has made the
way for me. When I meditate on His words, the command to love
more, I instantly think, "How?" How do I love You, Lord,

with all my heart and all my soul and all my mind? Might it be practicing the mighty five with You? The five love languages: words of affirmation, quality time, gifts, acts of service, and physical touch. Then, my God, I pray to praise You with my words daily, thanking You for all You have done and continue to do. I pray to spend more quality time with You, just You and I. And gifts . . . I will give You myself. My body will be Your temple and You do with it as You please. I will take care of this body and honor it because I belong to You. I will serve and take care of Your sheep. I will take care of those in front of me who need it the most . . . Yes, that is how I will serve You. Lastly, physical touch . . . this is a tough one for You, and I believe I have never seen You, nor have I ever touched You. But during my morning meditation, I sometimes imagine You taking my hand, holding me, and embracing me. So I will bring my thoughts back to this, Your tender touch and my resting beneath it. Father, as I practice loving You in all these ways, the second will come more easily because I will be filled with Your love. Father, I pray more of Your children learn how to participate in the

GREATEST COMMAND.

Jesus replied: "Love the Lord your God with all your heart and with all your soul and with all your mind." This is the first and greatest commandment. And the second is like it: "Love your neighbor as yourself."

Matthew 22:37-40 NIV

SOW WITH TEARS

God brings restoration and fortunes of all kinds—worldly fortunes and spiritual fortunes. All that is good comes from our Creator.

When I am in pain, I tend to forget this and ask, **WHY?** Why is this happening to me? There must be an easier way.

For every tear and ounce of pain you have ever experienced, God has more joy and blessing in store to triumph the pain.

You must trust His timeline. It's divine. He sees all things, and when you are ready, the songs of joy over your life will not be silenced.

Our Creator knows when you are ready . . . It's what makes the timeline so divine.

Dear Father, many many many tears I have shed. For a season of my life, that was all I knew. I cried until I dried, there were no more tears left in me, but that was the key! I had to walk through the pain, I had to let it do what it had come to do, let it change me. I could not fight it, so I surrendered to it and You exalted me. Lord, I pray for Your children all over the world today. I really want them to know that the tears they sow will be used to grow their space, land, and territory in this world. That the tears are good, healthy, and I encourage them to let them flow; fighting tears does us no good. Father, I want them to know when they are ready.

On Your divine timeline, there will be songs of joy that will not be silenced as they reap the harvest of all that grew from their tears. Lord, I pray more of us learn how to plant and *SOW WITH TEARS*.

Those who sow with tears will reap with songs of joy.

Psalm 126:5 NIV

DEPEND ON ME

What does it mean to depend on God? What does that look like?

Ask Him and wait for His answer
before you move.

Talk to Him, tell Him your thoughts,
and explain to Him how you feel.

Wait on Me
Hold on to Me
My words
My ways

Sometimes I feel torn. So torn it consumes me and I wrestle with
what I must do. When you really don't know how or what to do, ask
God and wait to act. Wait for His peace, His clarity.

It's all from Me, I go before you
Wait for Me before you move

Dear Lord, I have learned how to depend on You, so bountiful and
abundant are my fruits. You will produce many blessings for the
ones who learn and wait patiently for You. There are things You
have spoken to me that have passed and confirmed Your everlasting
promises, and there are things I am still waiting for, but it's the

dependence on You that brings these things to me. I pray for
Your children, may many more learn to lead a life that fully depends
on You. Lord, thank You for all the ways You have protected me
and shown me what I must do. It feels so much better living a life
where all does not
DEPEND ON ME.

But remember the LORD your God, for it is he who gives you the
ability to produce wealth, and so confirms his covenant.

Deuteronomy 8:18 NIV

NOTHING BEFORE ME

Why are you holding back?
There is enough room to love everything
I've put in your life—and fully
You are not protecting yourself by holding back on love, but
rather wasting space
Space that could be filled to create a more full life

God helps us love more, and when He is first, our
love is pure and complete. It's full and brings life
to areas that feel dead.

Vendy, I don't want anything else to come before Me
Nothing before Me
This isn't for Me, but for your protection
I'm the purest, My ways are higher and best

How do I put You first?

Trust, an everyday practice of surrender
Communication . . .
I am always here, always present, I see everything
I'm ready to listen

Dear God, Jesus said the most important command is to love You
with all our hearts and all our minds. It is to keep You first in our
daily ways and walk in obedience to You—that way we can walk in

Your true and good will. Lord, there have been nations that rose to rule in my life, making me feel like a small bug waiting to be smashed, but I clung to You and I walked away with the victory.

Navigating love, loss, death, losing a best friend, and swimming in the deep and cold waters, I'd like to name corporate America where they squeezed squeezed squeezed me! All these things have not overthrown me, and I look back with love, lots of love in my heart, because it was You Who got me through. Though I was drowning, I did not drown. Now it is You I aim to always keep first and not one thing, no

NOTHING BEFORE ME.

If you carefully observe all these commands I am giving you to follow—to love the LORD your God, to walk in obedience to him and to hold fast to him—then the LORD will drive out all these nations before you, and you will dispossess nations larger and stronger than you.

Deuteronomy 11:22-23 NIV

VICTORS WITH YOU

Regardless of the outcome, we can be victors with God.

You have to learn how to surrender the battle to Him.

Learning how to surrender has been the greatest and most challenging lesson of my life. One I continue to struggle with.

It's also the most rewarding and freeing thing a human can learn to do. When you surrender your circumstance to God, you are not giving up, you're displaying trust in Him. Trust that He has a way, a better solution or answer, that you cannot get to on your own.

Surrender is accepting that God, the all-powerful, not only knows what is around the corner, but has the power to go before you and make a way much better than anything you could have imagined.

Dear Lord, You have made me wise as a serpent and innocent as a dove. Because I have learned how to surrender my all to You, You send down Your angels to guard my steps and fight my battles. Swimming with sharks proves to be one less fear on my list as You have protected me in the midst of wolves. I pray for more of Your children to be
VICTORS WITH YOU.

Behold, I am sending you out as sheep in the midst of wolves, so be wise as serpents and innocent as doves.

Matthew 10:16 ESV

✦ LIKE ME ✦

I grow you to be like Me
Our hearts come together, and
you see the world through My eyes
People through My eyes
Situations through My eyes

God's goodness overflows, and once you experience it,
nothing else compares. You are filled with truth. Truth
that is freeing, truth that allows you to act and move in
ways that keep you blameless.

Dear Lord, thank You for blessing me with Your view. Instead of
grumbling, I waited for You to move. Purity in a crooked generation
is rare. I am ready to be placed in Your sky to shine brightly. I want
little ones to see those that cling to You, Your truth will shine,
they will be the brightest star in the sky
LIKE ME.

Do everything without grumbling or arguing, so that you may become blameless and pure,
"children of God without fault in a warped and crooked generation." Then you will shine
among them like stars in the sky as you hold firmly to the word of life.

Philippians 2:14-16 NIV

TODAY

Create a safe space for Me, set boundaries
around that second, minute, or hour
With practice, you will become stronger
and hear more from Me, sweet V

Create boundaries so you can learn how to be
present in the midst of life. There will always
be something new eating at you or running after
you. It's part of our ever-changing lives.

Dear God, thank You for blessing me with today. Help me,
please, create space in my mind and day for You. Please bless us
with the wisdom to choose You. When we choose a relationship with
You, filled with our time and Your loving presence, we slowly start
to hear from You. Father, for all Your children seeking and asking,
for all Your children that look to You, please give them
enough wisdom for
TODAY.

If any of you lacks wisdom, let him ask God, who
gives generously to all without reproach, and it
will be given Him.

James 1:5 ESV

LOVE AND CARE

Love and care, and you can never go wrong. When you do these two things without fear, you are successful wherever you go.

Care is the provision of what is necessary for the health, welfare, maintenance, and protection of someone or something.

Love is patient, kind, never proud or dishonoring, not easily angered, and keeps no record of wrongs.

When these two things become part of your soul, even when you get hurt for caring, you will never regret it. The key is to always place God first, that way your love and care stems from the purest place. When He is first, there's no such thing as a let down because your Creator will never let you down. 🩶

Dear Lord, when we look out for others' best interests, we create a peace-filled environment. When we treat one another with honor and respect, we become holy. God, it may not always be easy, which is why Your words instruct us to make every effort to love and care for one another. Some days this might be more challenging than others, but I pray to lead with more *LOVE AND CARE*.

Make every effort to live in peace with everyone and to be holy.

Hebrews 12:14 NIV

✦ *ALMIGHTY IN ME* ✦

Warrior: A brave or experienced soldier or fighter.

Brave: Showing courage.

🔑 Our Creator makes warriors.

Warriors against fear.
Warriors against anxiety.
Warriors against injustice.

But our hearts remain:
Pure 🤍
Gentle 🤍
Spotless 🤍

There is much to be done! Everyone's calling is different, but we all have a higher calling. There are daily battles, weekly battles, yearly battles, and lifetime battles.

🔑 We must understand that our Creator is always in control. Through the good and the bad.

🔑 When you make room for God's Spirit, He makes all things possible and the mightier His move.

Dear God, not by my might or power has my sweet and sassy 5'2" self been able to accomplish the many desires placed on my heart, but by and through Your Holy Spirit I have climbed to see victory!

It might not always take place the way I think it should, but that's because with You it's far better. I just wish I could learn to trust and be still long enough to wait on You. Wait on Your move! Faithful souls, please wait on the Lord. He weaves together plans for your life that require you to grow in Him; it won't happen the way you think it should because with God things are never how they seem! I love You, God, thank You for all You do and continue to do. May I continue to walk by faith and not by sight, for I have the

ALMIGHTY IN ME.

So he said to me, "This is the word of the Lord to Zerubbabel: 'Not by might nor by power, but by my Spirit,' says the Lord Almighty."

Zechariah 4:6 NIV

TOO WONDERFUL

God, are You able to do all things?
God, where are You now?
God, did You see what just happened?
God, I am starting to worry . . .
I don't understand how this could be?
God, can You hear me?
God, You told me to trust You!
God, why would You let this happen?
God, how do I keep trusting?

What is for you will not miss you if you are walking
in obedience and full surrender to Him.

There is so much we do not understand. Today I ask
God for a view from above. To help me navigate
from a place of knowledge, courage, love,
and hope.

Dear God, please help me to surrender. Help me hand my doubts
over to You, my fears, my anxieties, and all things that are after my
peace. You are too good and too wonderful for me to worry. Dear
God, help me to give it to You. Please send Your Spirit to lead me.
Let nothing come from my flawed, limited understanding, and let
my thoughts and actions be guided by Your Spirit because I don't
want to miss out on Your plans. They are just

TOO WONDERFUL.

I know that you can do all things; no purpose of yours can be thwarted. You
asked, "Who is this that obscures my plans without knowledge?" Surely I
spoke of things I did not understand, things too wonderful for me to know.

Job 42:2-3 NIV

JOY IN ME

God, help me to find joy in You so when my world feels like it is
falling apart, when things hurt me, I still have a strong sense of
peace because You are my foundation. In You, I have eternal joy
that lives in my heart.

Send up your request. Pray, ask, and seek
His peace and joy daily.

Dear Lord, please help me lay down and wait expectantly for You.
I love to wake to You each morning—it renews my hope, and I am
able to make it through another day. I am learning to have peace no
matter what is happening around me. Some days I feel fueled, some
days I am scared, some days I am hopeful, some days I am filled
with doubt, but the best days are always the ones where I turn to
You. No matter what I feel, as long as I wait for You, I am filled. I
love waking to You in the morning with my cup of matcha because it
sets my day and makes me new when I hear from You. Expectantly,
I wait for the Lord to move on my behalf, for the Lord to move
in me. I have peace, for He places
JOY IN ME!

In the morning, LORD, you hear my voice, in the morning
I lay my requests before you and wait expectantly.

Psalm 5:3 NIV

HEAVEN MINDSET

Vendy, although I was God . . . I lived in a human body

Flesh and blood limits you. The key is
having a heaven mindset.

Know there will be pain and suffering, but understand it's not for us
to take on the brokenness in this world or always understand why it
takes place.

Vendy, I did not come to take it away but to make a way
To give hope and peace to you while you are in the midst of this
broken world is what I do

You can't take on the brokenness of the
world. You can't let it enter your mind
and heart—otherwise it will overcome you.

We are called to be transformed by our spirits, so we do not conform
to the ways of this world.

God will give you a view from above.
He will teach you how to love others
no matter what and to understand that it's not
a battle between flesh and blood but spiritual
forces of evil in the heavenly
realms opposing love.

Dear Lord, Prince of Peace, Messiah, Immanuel, Lamb of God, Light of the World, and King of Kings, thank You for leaving heaven and the Father to rescue me. If You would have never left His right hand and entered this broken world, this girl would not have had a way. Thank You for lifting a very heavy cross and laying down Your innocent life for a spoiled, impatient child like me. I don't understand the brokenness I see, but with You, Jesus, I really don't need to because You do it. You did the deed and now my heart and mind are guarded with Your truth. It's the only thing that will ever set the captives free! Jesus, thank You for leaving Your kingdom filled with armies of angels to come and be with me. I do not deserve You or what You have done, but I will try to live a life that honors You. I will try to be Your hands and feet, taking steps and shaking hands with people who share this

HEAVEN MINDSET.

And the peace of God, which surpasses all understanding,
will guard your hearts and your minds in Christ Jesus.

Philippians 4:7 ESV

MY STRENGTH AND SONG

Oh, Vendy, the ways I protect you. I wish you could see
The times, the signs, all from Me 🤍

Mornings are my favorite because it's the most protected time I have. The time where I get to be with You and not think about anything else. Or if I am thinking of something else, You give me peace. Lord, I love you. I miss spending more time with You, and I just want to be with You.

There will be many different seasons of life, but time with God is always something you can count on. He is always there.

Dear Lord, quiet the waves in this busy season. You have displayed my strength, and it is not in me but You, which means, Lord, I need more time with You. But this season is very busy, so what must I do? Take You with me? Throughout my day? How? I would love to, but the morning is the only time I can be still and focus on You. Ask You to come with me? Join me in my day, invite Your Spirit to drive with me to work, to open my laptop and watch me type away? Ohhh, time and time again You have given me the victory by whispering the way. So yes, of course, I will try this today! Lord, please send Your Holy Spirit to work with me, please don't leave my side, and be *MY STRENGTH AND SONG.*

The Lord is my strength and my song;
he has given me victory.

Exodus 15:2 NLT

ALL IN MY HANDS

God, I need a day filled with peace. A day from You, Lord. Open my eyes and help me see the everyday blessings. It really is You I love, and only You have the ability to help me see.

Stress
Fear
Anxiety
Bow to me—you have no authority over me.

The blood has been shed, and He says walk free, so you must flee.

Dear Lord, please help me place my fears, worries, doubts, confusions, and distress in Your hands, and help me release
ALL IN MY HANDS.

But will God really dwell on earth with humans? The heavens, even the highest heavens, cannot contain you.

2 Chronicles 6:18 NIV

RUN IN YOUR PATH

I want to be close to Your heartbeat, to love You more and more with every day that passes.

Thank You, Lord, for the good and the bad. The good has made my life so sweet. The bad has brought me closer to You and revealed Your goodness.

🔑 Thank God for all He has done
and continues to do. 🤍

Dear God, I pray for greater faith, courage, and love. I pray for more of Your Spirit and less of me. I pray for Your will to surround the surface of this world. 🌍 Help me sprint in the path of Your commands. May I never grow tired, for I always want to
RUN IN YOUR PATH!

I run in the path of your commands, for
you have broadened my understanding.

Psalm 119:32 NIV

MY FAITHFULNESS

Our Creator loves justice. It is through His faithfulness that we see justice in areas of our lives. Not because we deserve it or because we have done anything to win it in a broken world, but because God's hand is on it!

When things don't feel fair in my life, I have a hard time trusting God.

All I know is God loves justice, no will of His can be thwarted, and it's through His faithfulness that we see justice.

Dear God, please help me to see how You see, give me a view from above that transcends my understanding. Give me strength and purpose to move exactly how You see fit. Direct each step and bless me with Your peace. Not because I deserve it, but because of Your faithfulness. Lift Your children up all around the world who do right by You. May the fruits of their gardens be seen and shine bright in the light of day—for the righteous deserve the praise! My God, I love You and desire to do right by You because You have always done right by me. I know I will fail, but please strengthen *MY FAITHFULNESS.*

For as the soil makes the sprout come up and a garden causes seeds to grow, so the Sovereign LORD will make righteousness and praise spring up before all nations.

Isaiah 61:11 NIV

MY WAVES, MY WAYS

I love all My people
I am constantly moving
I am constantly loving
I am constantly choosing you
You can have peace at any and
every moment of your life with Me
It's a choice
You can choose to trust Me
Choose to believe that
I'm here . . . listening and fighting
on your behalf
Or you can choose to not

Trust is like a muscle; faith grows with
practice. But it's always a choice.

Sweet V, I follow you
I love you and
I just want you to choose Me
When you choose Me, you reach higher
When you choose Me, no eye has seen all that I can do
No eye
Choose Me every day, every moment, and every time
And watch Me move

Dear Lord, I crave Your waves, so I must choose Your ways! You have gotten me this far, and because I choose You, my steps are ordered and placed on grounds all from You. My Holy Father, I really love You. Please grow my faith muscle so I can do mighty things and cause the world to look to You. Or maybe I don't do mighty things, but I pray to live in a world where more souls turn to You. Father, we need more of You, so lessen

MY WAVES, MY WAYS.

Who, then, are those who fear the LORD? He will
instruct them in the ways they should choose.

Psalm 25:12 NIV

CLOSE YOUR EYES & OPEN YOUR HEART

We are called to act out of a place of faith. We move, trust, and take a step forward—not knowing the outcome. Faith is blind, and I have such a hard time acting from a place of faith.

What does it look like to open my heart?
Love and serve.

Dear God, close my eyes and open my heart 🤍 so that no plan of Yours can be thwarted. So that rivers of life will flow from my life. Father, I believe I have seen Your hand move in my life in ways beyond my wildest dreams, and yet I struggle to have faith in the unseen. Help me love and serve who You would like me to love and serve. Please whisper to me, give me the keys, tell me . . . *Sweet V, CLOSE YOUR EYES & OPEN YOUR HEART.*

Anyone who believes in me may come and drink! For the
Scriptures declare, "Rivers of living water will
flow from his heart."

John 7:38 NLT

GOD'S WILL

To know My heart
To know how much I care
To know My love

I write to God, I pray to God, and I spend time with God, yet I'm
so quick to forget His guidance. But if there is one thing that never
fails me, it's the knowledge of God's love. This understanding is
powerful because no human, career, or earthly matter can
offer you something . . .

So consistent and full
So permanent and beautiful
So pure and simple

God's will for every human is to know the
depths of His love because in His love, we
find identity and truth that empowers us.

When we have peace, God is happy.
Our peace makes the Creator of
all things happy.

Dear Father, I pray Your will be done on earth as it is in heaven. The
scary part of this prayer is there is a chance Your will might not be
done. Your Son instructs us to pray that the Father's will be done on

earth. God, I pray for more of Your creation to know Your heart, to know how much You care, to know it's Your love that has the power to create the most beautiful version of their lives if they would just accept Your love. Lord, I pray for more hearts and souls to pray *GOD'S WILL.*

For wisdom will enter your heart, and knowledge
will be pleasant to your soul.

Proverbs 2:10 NIV

GUIDING LIGHT

Vendy, hold in your heart a special place for Me
That way you will always have a guiding light
And with that light, you will never get lost

On our worst days, He is still so good.
His character is pure, true, and loving.

Dear God, thank You for blessing me with this beautiful life. One full of love and light because of You. Thank You for my family, friends, coworkers, and all the good that happens daily that I fail to recognize. My dear Lord, I pray to always be Yours. Help me, Lord, place all my trust in You. Today I feel I am being pushed, spread too thin, and I might break if You do not move soon. I am trying to run and hold on to the space in my heart for You because I really could use Your light. Please, Father, I need Your light to shine so I don't get lost or stray from Your path. Help me place my hope in You all day long, for You are my
GUIDING LIGHT.

Show me your ways, Lord, teach me your paths. Guide me in your
truth and teach me, for you are God my Savior, and my hope is in
you all day long.

Psalm 25:4-5 NIV

NOTHING I DON'T TOUCH

There is nothing God does not see because He is omnipresent:
present everywhere at the same time.

If we believe this about God's nature, then we do our best to honor
Him in our relationships, our work, and all areas of our lives because
God sees it all. Even if the outcome is not always fair or how you'd
like it to be, God is present and sees your every move.

God has the power to touch our mouths, minds,
hearts, and wills, so His words, thoughts, love,
and actions are in us.

Dear Lord, stretch out Your hand and place Your words in my
mouth. Fill my mind with Your thoughts and give me Your feet to
steer my path, for I am growing weak and tired—oh so tired—of
doing good! I really need Your help because of all I see, Lord. I need
help honoring, I need help believing that there is not a single part of
my life that Your Holy hand does not cover. I must believe this so I
have peace and can honor those who do not honor me; I know it is
really for You and there is nothing I would not do for You. Father,
help me believe and still me so I can just be. Let it all be You. Keep
me and my flesh out of the way and tell me, *Sweet V, there is
NOTHING I DON'T TOUCH.*

Then the LORD stretched out His hand and touched my mouth, and the
LORD said to me, "Behold, I have put My words in your mouth."

Jeremiah 1:9 NASB

YOUR SAVIOR

The power of God's truth has moved in my life when
I needed it most.

Great is our Creator's faithfulness.

You have brought me so far, knowing exactly when to withhold
or grant me a sign of encouragement.

Dear Lord, thank You for making the way. You have never led me
astray—even when I passed through the waters, the fire did not
burn me and the water did not overcome me. Today as I write to
You, lacking oh so much faith, I need You to remind me of Your
faithfulness. I need You to remind me that You are not a limited
human with a limited view and a weak will, but an all-powerful
God Who breathed me to life and knows every detail of my life.
For all of us, may we recall who suffered the most injustice of all,
the blameless Lamb Who had an army of angels at His command,
yet laid down His life so we may be free. When I want to complain
or my lack of faith gets in the way, remind me of the Son You sent.
Remind us all of
YOUR SAVIOR.

Do not fear, for I have redeemed you; I have summoned you by name; you are mine.
When you pass through the waters, I will be with you; and when you pass through the
rivers, they will not sweep over you. When you walk through the fire, you will not be
burned; the flames will not set you ablaze. For I am the LORD your God, the Holy One
of Israel, your Savior.

Isaiah 43:1-3 NIV

FEBRUARY

PEACE

Lord, time with You is the only thing that gives me peace nowadays.
Maybe it's what I just walked through, maybe it's what I am walking
through, or maybe it's what happens when we grow close to You.
Your ways are so different, so much higher; it hurts because we
see how far this world is from You.

Pray for more of God and less of you.

Dear Lord, help me to enjoy the ride. The waves, the crashing
on the shore, the reflection of the sun, the cool from the night. Help
me to enjoy the ride, Lord. Help me to be grateful. I know I have so
much to be grateful for, yet I forget and continue to reason using
my own logic. Logic that falls so short compared to
Your wisdom and ways. Lord, be my
PEACE.

Now may the Lord of peace himself give you peace at all
times and in every way. The Lord be with all of you.

2 Thessalonians 3:16 NIV

MY DAD

No matter the weather,
your dad always had joy, Vendy

These past few days I've been missing my dad more than ever.
Reflecting on the memories I have with him brings me comfort; he
feels less distant when I think of the twenty-three years
we had together.

I'm missing my father's love, his touch, and time with him. Things
I will never experience again on earth.

I'm especially missing his joyful spirit. No matter the situation, he
had joy. He brought joy to those he cared for because he was so
lighthearted. His heart was childlike in many ways.

This world is temporary, and living with a
carefree, childlike heart is what God
desires for our lives.

How do we do this when it's rainy? Or cold? Or windy?

We trust God, we draw close and relax there.
We breathe there. And communicate our
hearts to Him. The Creator. Then we are ready
to step back in. To face the world no
matter the weather.

Dear God, what brings me peace with his passing is simple: knowing it was his time. His time to go. His time for complete peace. His time for complete love. His time for eternal joy. His time to be taken care of. His time for rest, unlike anything we will ever experience on earth. God, Your heart was ready for my dad and that's a peace I have that transcends all. 🤍 🙏 He will never be forgotten, and his love lives on and through me . . . I will forever miss *MY DAD*.

And the peace of God, which transcends all understanding,
will guard your hearts and your minds in Christ Jesus.

Philippians 4:7 NIV

LITTLE FAITH

Do we truly believe on our worst days how good God is?
His true nature?

We will have good days, we will have bad days, and God is always
there. He is always moving.

If God can control the wind, the wind
that has no master, what do you think
He can do in your life? What do you
think He can control or make happen in
your life?

Dear God, I am of such little faith, please open my eyes. Even the
wind and waves obey Your voice, Your voice that greets me every
morning, and yet I find myself feeding my fears rather than my faith!
Oh, me of little faith. My God, You Who calms the waves and makes
a way. Please grow my faith, help me rely on Your ways more, Lord.
Even as I write these words to You, Father, I am filled with doubt,
which I know hurts You. Help me laugh at the future and all that
comes against the Almighty's will for me. Oh, silly me of
LITTLE FAITH.

He got up and ordered the wind to stop. He said to the waves, "Quiet! Be still!" Then the
wind died down. And it was completely calm. He said to his disciples, "Why are you so
afraid? Don't you have any faith at all yet?" They were terrified. They asked each other,
"Who is this? Even the wind and the waves obey him!"

Mark 4:39-41 NIRV

JUST BELIEVE

Afraid: Worried that something undesirable will occur
or be done.

What is causing you fear? Why is it causing you fear?

Ask yourself, "What is truth?" What is getting in the way of that
truth? Is it fear of what could happen? Fear of the unknown?

Ask God to help you do what is right and
lay down what is wrong.

*It is in My hands, so I need you to
trust Me and believe, Vendy*

Dear Lord, help me
JUST BELIEVE.

Overhearing what they said, Jesus told him,
"Don't be afraid; just believe."

Mark 5:36 NIV

NATIONS LARGER

Vendy, your ability to hear from Me
depends on how much you choose Me daily
How much you shut out the world
and other voices, and wait on Me
Talk to Me
Give to Me

It is in that quiet space where you will hear
from God and His will becomes clear.

This world is not just, and
you will not always see justice take place
But if you keep My ways,
I will guard your heart and mind
And you will dispossess nations larger
and stronger than you
Giants in your life will fall
and I will do great things through you

Dear Lord, I love You with my whole heart. I try my hardest to be
obedient to Your Holy Spirit and I cling to You, especially when
I am conflicted. I am ready to see You move on my behalf, Lord.

I would like to see the nations larger than me bend a knee to Your ways. I would like to see You drive out the evil at play in my life, and wherever You take me next, may it be fully mine. Lord, the training is almost complete for me! The heavens are shouting for joy because I am ready for the ones much greater than I, the *NATIONS LARGER.*

If you carefully observe all these commands I am giving you to follow—to love the LORD your God, to walk in obedience to him and to hold fast to him—then the LORD will drive out all these nations before you, and you will dispossess nations larger and stronger than you. Every place where you set your foot will be yours.

Deuteronomy 11:22-24 NIV

HELP ME TRUST

Sometimes we feel hurt by friends, family, work, or situations in this world.

What helps me most is knowing that there is
an all-powerful God working things out on
my behalf. Our Creator is weaving together both
the good and the bad events in your life for
your greater good!

Dear God, please help me to trust You. Help me follow You. Bless me, grow me, protect me so I can stay on Your path, walk in Your will, go where You'd like me to go. Bless me with Your peace to love and serve. Bless the work of my hands with Your faithful and just ways, but only if You see fit. Father,
HELP ME TRUST.

He has shown his people the power of his works, giving them the lands
of other nations. The works of his hands are faithful and just; all his
precepts are trustworthy. They are established for ever and ever,
enacted in faithfulness and uprightness.

Psalm 111:6-8 NIV

SOMETHING NEW

I will never want anything but Your will because I know Your nature, truth, beauty, and power. You are the only One I want to serve. You, my dear Lord, are the only just One.

God will show you what you need to be grateful for and who to pray for; all we must do is ask.

Dear Lord, help me to walk in Your will. I don't want anything that pulls me away. Close every door You want me to avoid, those that will take me away from Your will. Open and allow only Your desire for my life—keep me out of the way, for I know nothing, and it's You that created me! You have loved and nursed me back to life, the old is gone and now there is *SOMETHING NEW.*

Therefore, if anyone is in Christ, the new creation
has come: The old has gone, the new is here!

2 Corinthians 5:17 NIV

YOUR HEART

Our hearts ♡ are shaped by life events. Ones that test us and grow us.

Allow God to shape your heart through your life events by trusting He is in control.

We live in a broken world and pain is part of this world. 🌑 Anytime we do not choose His ways, pain is an outcome of not choosing the light.

What He does through the pain is great: We grow and are tested through faith. When we trust Him through life events, we allow God to shape and mold our hearts ♥ into life-giving sources. Ones that are strong, courageous, and honorable.

Dear Lord, help me to love You with all my strength, mind, and soul. Shape my heart to be like
YOUR HEART.

Love the LORD your God with all your heart and with all your soul and with all your mind and with all your strength.

Mark 12:30 NIV

FEARFUL

Fear: An unpleasant emotion caused by the belief that someone or something is dangerous, likely to cause pain, or a threat.

Fear is caused by a belief.

What do you choose to believe?

I don't want you to be fearful
When you have fear, you are not trusting
that I am with you
The Creator of all things, the all-powerful God
Who goes before you

The opposite of fear is faith.

When you are with Me there is no fear
Bring Me with you today, everywhere you go
More of My Spirit = less fear

Dear Lord, I am Your faithful one. I ask that You protect me and all Your faithful children who are navigating their way through deep waters. I ask that You send Your Holy Spirit to guide us wherever we go today, even if it's just downstairs to the kitchen for a cup of water! And, Father, whoever of Your faithful children are struggling with fear, please let them know that You are with them, for them, and You are near. Let them know You will honor them who have so desperately tried to honor You. Let them know that the things they love—their family, friends, hopes, dreams—are all secure and safely resting with You today. Let them move forward with the strength and courage of a lion. Let them be gentle, kind, honest, courageous, and no longer

FEARFUL.

For he guards the course of the just and protects the way of his faithful ones.

Proverbs 2:8 NIV

AGAPE DAY

Valentine's Day: A holiday where lovers express their affection with greetings and gifts, and at the end of the fifth century, it came to be celebrated as a day of romance.

There is a love in my life and it's different than any love I've ever felt before. This love has always been there, I've just never poured into it the way I do now.

I look forward to one day sharing my life with someone, every part of it, every part of me, but I know the love I experience from another human relationship will never be able to do what this love does and has done for me.

This love keeps me going, it lights my steps and makes my heart 🤍 full.

Our Creator is love. He turns the lights on in complete darkness. He speaks life over and into you. He is always there and never stops caring.

This is a perfect love because God is perfect.

This love is agape love. 🤍 The highest form of love.

Dear Lord, reflecting on love today, I'm grateful for all the areas in my life where I experience it, but I'm especially grateful for the love I've received from above. This love has moved mountains and continues to give me life. It's one I will have forever and one that is free to every human. This love is the most powerful source in my life, and I'm just so grateful to have my eyes open to this love. You, Lord, it's You. You keep my lamp burning, and with You, my darkness becomes light! So today I celebrate You, my love, on this

AGAPE DAY.

You, LORD, keep my lamp burning; my God turns my darkness into light.

Psalm 18:28 NIV

HOLD YOUR HEART

Happiness. What does it mean to be happy?

Happy: Feeling or showing pleasure or contentment.

Contentment: A state of satisfaction.

God wants our days to be full and filled with joy. I don't want to be content. I want to be thriving. But I get confused as to what that looks like.

Some days I am stressed, some days are slow, some days I just want to go for a walk or see a movie, some days I want to be with my friends and I crave excitement. Some days I confuse myself and do the opposite of what my body or spirit needs.

God, how do I achieve happiness when each day is different?

Just ask God what you need more of
each day, and then ask for His help
in getting there.

Dear Lord, today what do I need more of? Show me, help me make the right choice. Help me be grateful. Help me choose You and Your peace. Your law, statutes, and precepts are perfectly trustworthy, so I hand my heart, life, and soul over to You. Show me just what I need each day, and, Father, show me how I can love You better too! I want to give joy to more hearts. I want to be more like You. My God, I love the way You give to me, it refreshes my soul and makes my simple ways wise. Please, Lord, promise me You will forever and always be with me on earth to hold me like You did when my dear Al passed. Promise me, Lord, You will always do this for me, and I promise You, God, whoever You send to me, under my care and watch, I will do my best to hold their heart the way He holds our hearts. The one and only Son. He is the one Who taught us, and His heart is the one that belonged to You. It is only through the Son that we will be able to get to the heart of the Father. Only through the Son will we be able to

HOLD YOUR HEART.

The law of the LORD is perfect, refreshing the soul. The statutes of the LORD are trustworthy, making wise the simple. The precepts of the LORD are right, giving joy to the heart.

Psalm 19:7-8 NIV

WAKE UP WITH ME

Waking up with Me gives new hope and energizes your life

My favorite part of each day is waking up and spending time with God. It is a time where I feel most clear and at peace. My mornings and time spent with my Creator have brought me through loss and any life challenges that arise.

I wish I could spend my entire day with the feeling I get in the morning after spending time with Him. As I move throughout my day, sometimes the clarity I received so powerfully in the a.m. fades, and the motion of life takes over.

He refreshes our souls; we just need to give
Him a little of our time.

Dear Lord, thank You for my mornings and moments with You. May they always be the highlight ☀ of my life. God, help me to bring the peace You give me each morning with me throughout my day. I pray more souls gain a hunger to wake to You each morning. I pray they experience what I have been so greatly blessed with—a desire for time with You. For Your name's sake, You have refreshed my soul, and I pray You always
WAKE UP WITH ME.

He makes me lie down in green pastures, he leads me beside quiet
waters, he refreshes my soul. He guides me along the right
paths for his name's sake.

Psalm 23:2-3 NIV

FUMBLE WITH ME

When we start something new, we are not always good at it.
Sometimes it takes a while for us to catch on, sometimes God
allows us to go through the bumpy parts before calming the water.
Sometimes the water stays the same, but He better equips us.

God doesn't care if you fumble. What matters
is that you do it with Him.

There is no losing with God because He uses it all. Sometimes it just
takes a minute to get over the hump, to turn the corner and see all
He is doing.

Dear God, please help me place my hope in You every day. Not
just on the bad days or the good days, but every day. My God,
guard my life and rescue me, fill me with Your wisdom, and do not
let my name be put to shame because I trust and seek You, Lord.
May my steps always be directed by You, dripping in integrity and
honor because it is You I hope in. It is You Who fights my battles.
It is You Who goes before me. It is You Who weaves together my
wildest dreams. Oh, Father, please never leave my side. I know I will
continue to trip, but it is You Who stays near, picks me back up. You
FUMBLE WITH ME.

Guard my life and rescue me; do not let me be put to shame, for
I take refuge in you. May integrity and uprightness protect me,
because my hope, LORD, is in you.

Psalm 25:20-21 NIV

SECURITY OF MY LIFE

The Bible speaks a lot on fear. It tells us not to fear ever because
God did not give us a spirit of fear.

Fear is removed in my life when I trust in
God's true nature and place His ways first.

If you **KNOW** the most powerful source, the Creator of all things, is
where your hope, strength, and joy stems from, then . . . if you truly
believe this, which is very hard because we live in such a broken
world, it is impossible for you to ever go wrong.

If you **KNOW** and believe this about God, then the second step
is placing Him at the center. When God is your stronghold
(a place of security), it doesn't matter what happens to or around
you because you are standing on solid ground.

If you can do these two things, then fear will not overcome you. As
I have experienced many times, fear only holds you back, causes
anxiety, or stops you from obtaining
all God has for you.

What do I fear? What is my stronghold?
What in my life is my light?

Dear God, light of my life, thank You for breaking chains and
causing the infamous fear in my life to bow. My God, there is
nothing more powerful than You, and as a result, growing closer
to You caused me to grow in power! The fear that once lived in my
bones and occupied my mind no longer has a stronghold in me.
Yes, it took much suffering, many tears, and a series of humbling
things to break me, but the breaking created something new. It
broke off the fear and made me into something like You!
Divine I am because You are the
SECURITY OF MY LIFE.

The LORD is my light and my salvation—whom shall I fear? The
LORD is the stronghold of my life—of whom shall I be afraid?

Psalm 27:1-2 NIV

GOD'S VOICE

How can I hear more of God's voice? This powerful,
majestic voice . . .

God is moving in every human's life; we are His creation. Some
people choose to see His movement and others choose not to.

The key to recognizing God's voice, His Spirit
at play in your life, is thanking Him for all
He has done, and choosing Him each day.

When you ascribe glory to God, chains break.

God doesn't need our praise. He doesn't need the credit; it's for our
own benefit. It's for our own guidance and strength . . . So choose
God, and your ears and heart will be open to the power.

Dear Lord, my Creator of all, I pray more of Your children come
running to You! I know if more people walking this earth heard
from You, we would live in a much more whole world. My God,
my sweet Lord, I do not deserve Your goodness, but I welcome it.
I embrace it because it is Your powerful, majestic voice I have
learned to wake to. Oh, King of Kings, I pray more souls bend a
knee to You at the sound of Your voice. For what could
possibly be mightier than
GOD'S VOICE?

The voice of the LORD is powerful; the voice of the LORD is majestic.

Psalm 29:4 NIV

GENERATIONS

The more you see yourself the way God sees you, the more you will be able to do. Great blessings will stem from your life for generations to come.

How do we see ourselves the way God sees us when we spend the majority of our time with coworkers, friends, or family?

You must choose to make time for Him.

Dear God, help me to see myself the way You see me. Help me to not place my identity in things that may fail me, fade, or lack foundation. Help me, Lord, to choose You. God, what are the purposes of Your heart for me? I want to see them come to be. I want to walk in Your plans because they bring blessings not only to me and all I love, but generations to come. How is that a thing? Because You are the mighty Creator of all Who stands firm forever for generations on *GENERATIONS*.

But the plans of the LORD stand firm forever, the purposes of his heart through all generations.

Psalm 33:11 NIV

MY HAND

I'm not sure if God has a hand large enough for me, but if He does, I'd like to rest in it. With a view from above.

When you rest in Me
When you find hope in Me
When you believe Me, you are free to be yourself,
who I created you to be in My image
Not the image the world places on you, wrapping you in chains
of fear, stress, worry, or lies

What is for you truly is in God's hands. It's important to believe and trust this so we can . . .

Enjoy today. Be present to the many blessings of today.

Lead with love because we feel safe and cared for.

God offers a way always. It's up to us to choose it each and every day, especially in the middle of trying times.

Dear Lord, there have been times when the hand of the wicked came oh so close to getting the best of me. But since I choose to rest in Your hand, my ways mark You and they are not able to get to me. My ways are filled with wisdom because I wait on You, I rely on

You and not all I see, which oftentimes deceives me! But You, Who
are wise and have a view from above, direct me. Who can catch me
when You are the One that defends me? My God, thank You
for leading the way and holding
MY HAND.

May the foot of the proud not come against me,
nor the hand of the wicked drive me away.

Psalm 36:11 NIV

DELIGHT IN ME

Because He created us, He planted certain desires in our
hearts. 💕 He planted dreams, people, family members,
and hopes in our lives.

My fullest life, your fullest life, happens when the
Creator's vision for us comes true.

The more His creation submits to and walks in
His will, the more fulfilled desires we will see.

Dear Lord, You know the desires of my heart more than me. You
are the One that created me, blessed me with certain gifts and
weaknesses. The gifts I have are wonderful, for they point to You.
My weaknesses . . . well, they are great too, for they keep me
clinging to You! I have been afflicted and brought to my knees, and
at one point in my life it was a daily thing—the many many tears
I shed. But, everyone, take hope, for these afflictions are what cause
me to take delight in You, my Lord. And now that I truly delight in
You, the desires You planted deep in me will all come to be, so
I pray pray pray more of Your creation learns to delight in You!
For You are the One Who places
DELIGHT IN ME.

Take delight in the LORD, and he will give you
the desires of your heart.

Psalm 37:4 NIV

MY WINDOW

God, I'm thankful for my window. I'm thankful for waking up each
morning to the green banana trees, soft ocean breeze, and
blue sky.

Lord, I'm grateful for my large window. It brings me so much peace
in the morning, waking up to Your creation. So simple, but
I love my window.

I know I won't have this window forever. The view
will change, maybe I'll have a larger window
one day . . . but for right now, I'm so thankful for this
window, this view. Oh, the mighty things that
gratitude can do!

Dear God, I have looked out this window in my little room in
Playa del Rey by the sea day after day. And although my view has
not changed, I see this window oh so differently today because I am
filled with gratitude. It's a beautiful thing for us to learn how to draw
close to You. When we learn what it looks like to seek You each day,
You change our view. Even if my window is the same, You gave
me new eyes to see it differently. For one day, I will live in a home
with a family of my own, and this little room with a window by the
sea will not be what I see. This time will never come again, so thank
You, my God, for opening my eyes today and helping me see
MY WINDOW.

I will give thanks to you, LORD, with all my heart.

Psalm 9:1 NIV

TODAY

Because our hearts and souls were created for eternity, this world has a powerful ability to make you feel like there is something more you should be doing. But the truth is, there will always be a big empty space in your heart as long as you find meaning in things of this world.

Reflecting on my life this morning, I realize that there is not one desire, dream, or thing that could happen to me today that would bring more joy to my life than the joy I have already found in God.

Why?

Because things of this world are not meant to last forever, but God does, love does, and His love lasts forever . . . and that's about it.

As you reach new heights in your life and your dreams come true, as you journey through different stages of your life, no matter how great the height or dream, it will never be enough. There will always be pain and suffering in this world. 🌑 There will always be something else to cross off your list.

God shapes the desires and fires of our hearts so as they change, similar to the way this world changes, God will be at the center and we can find meaning, joy, and purpose in each stage of life. The waiting, the fulfillment, and everything in between.

Dear Lord, I will never be more happy today than I will tomorrow or with anything You bless me with because I know, I truly know, that my happiness, my joy, and my peace are found in You. And I have access to You at any and every moment of my life. So, God, I pray to always choose You. My God, I desire Your will all my days—not just

TODAY!

I desire to do your will, my God; your law is within my heart.

Psalm 40:8 NIV

MARCH

GOD AS YOUR GUIDE

When I allow God to be my guide, I have peace. I don't always choose Him or His ways; I get stuck thinking I know best . . . but when that fails me, I call on Him and He has a way of making everything better, regardless of the mess I created.

God allows love to be our guide
when He is by our side.

Ask God what specifically you
need guidance on today.

Dear Lord, as I navigate the twists and turns of life, I pray to call upon Your love to be my ultimate guide. Father, Your children, all of Your children, let them know today that they cannot go wrong with the Creator of the universe as their guide. Lord, the Son, the one Who came, died, and rose from the grave, He said it was You! You Who acted as His guide, and He promised to send His Spirit. I know this is true because I have experienced the guidance of the Holy Spirit. I have experienced God as my guide and so did He. He spoke oftentimes of what a life looked like with
GOD AS YOUR GUIDE.

For this God is our God for ever and ever;
he will be our guide even to the end.

Psalm 48:14 NIV

HUNGER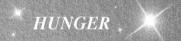

What creates a hunger for the Lord?

What creates a steadfast spirit?

Steadfast: Dutifully firm and unwavering.

I usually desire more of God when things are going wrong. I'm learning to praise, love, and be with Him more simply because it feeds me and brings me joy, but it's much easier to spend time with Him when things are not going as I would like. When I'm confused or don't know what to do.

This is part of our journey. The unknown is a tool used to bring us closer, similar to pain and suffering. They can all be used to bring us closer to our Creator.

Dear Lord, create a pure heart in me so I can love who You want me to love, serve You through the good and the bad, and desire You more than I desire anything of this world. Feed me with Your courage. Lions, You create, because for You we *HUNGER*.

Create in me a pure heart, O God, and
renew a steadfast spirit within me.

Psalm 51:10 NIV

MY FORTRESS

I remember how painful it was when my dad passed. I don't remember all the days filled with tears, but I remember the pain of it. I remember waking up, needing God.

Now, I don't always wake up and feel like I need God. But I do wake up and know what He has done. I remember my many early mornings—lighting a candle, watching the sun rise, and feeling held. Held together. I don't fully understand it, but I was able to find so much comfort in the midst of so much pain, because God was holding me.

I love my mornings, but they are not fully the same. I now realize what a beautiful thing it is to need and experience God's comfort.

Our Creator is close to the brokenhearted,
and though we will heal and move
forward, the true strength lies in knowing
where your power comes from.
Where your fortress lies.

Dear Lord, I now know my power; I now have the key! I am a young woman who may be tempted and tested, but because You are the One I turn to, I am not as susceptible to outside influence or disturbance. You are my strength . . . Oh, thank You for being *MY FORTRESS*.

You are my strength, I watch for you; you, God,
are my fortress, my God on whom I can rely.

Psalm 59:9-10 NIV

LOSE HEART

How do we avoid losing heart?

Sometimes I must remind myself of what God has already done in my life. Because of what He has already done through His Son and the many blessings I have, I can remain hopeful for all the beauty that is ahead.

Only God has the power to renew us day by day.

Our troubles are **ALL** momentary, and they will be far outweighed by what God has in store. If you know and believe this, you can always get back up each day.

Dear Lord, I am a young woman with a healthy body, and although it might not always be that way—my body will one day waste away and crumble to old age—inwardly You have the power to renew. Both the light and momentary troubles I experience on earth do not compare to the daily beauty and glory that lives in Your kingdom, which is built for eternity unlike this fallen world. But, Father, while I am here, keep me strong in You. You make me courageous. Please, God, protect me. Never do I want to *LOSE HEART.*

Therefore we do not lose heart. Though outwardly we are wasting away, yet inwardly we are being renewed day by day. For our light and momentary troubles are achieving for us an eternal glory that far outweighs them all.

2 Corinthians 4:16-17 NIV

NOT WELCOMED

Yes, God can do anything. He is all-powerful and can do whatever He wants.

We also have power. We are created in His image, and in Jesus' name we have authority to cast away unwanted spirits.

Fear and anxiety, you are not welcome here.

God is never late. Sometimes His delay can be
for us—for a true realization of our own
power . . . the power His Son freely
gave to us.

Dear God, as I have ventured to new heights, I have been greeted by new demons of all types. Anxiety, fear, and pride . . . oh, the mighty ways they were after me. Many nights I lost sleep, could not eat, but they did not win. Rather, they gave me the keys to unlock my victory. Prayer, worship music, matcha lattes, and time with You was what kept me! The worship music made them cry, they hated it and did not know how to scream their lies over the truth that flowed from my tunes! The longer my prayers, the louder the music, and stronger my lattes, they knew I was here to stay, and they were no longer welcomed. They no longer had authority over me because I knew how to fight the hidden things that we do not see. The eye deceives, but the soul knows. The soul craves truth, and the flesh's needs must outweigh the soul's goals! Oh, Father, I have my secret sauce, my delightful recipe to fight these demons and forever make them flee me! They run and with them take their lies. My Lord, my deliverer, thank You for casting them away. I pray You enlighten the hurting minds and struggling souls who do not even know what they are battling today! They do not even know what is happening in their everyday lives. Father, teach them how to fight the king of lies, for he is

NOT WELCOMED.

You are my help and my deliverer;
LORD, do not delay.

Psalm 70:5 NIV

WORTHY

God doesn't want us to worry. He wants us to know we are taken
care of. All is taken care of.

What could this look like?

It's the peace in finding joy and pleasure in
life's simplest things. Sunset walks, a cup
of coffee, a delicious taco, a hug from a friend,
a call from a loved one, a smile from a stranger,
a candy-painted sky, a restful Sunday . . . whatever
it may be.

You are worthy of joy in the most simple and
abundant ways. God loves people so much.
He never wants us to live in fear or worry.

Dear God, please help me to be like the birds in the sky. To soar high
above my fears, to fly in the colorful sky, to enjoy Your creation, to
live high, dwelling close to the heavens and You. For I know, more
than the birds in the sky, I am
WORTHY.

Look at the birds in the sky! They don't plant or harvest. They don't
even store grain in barns. Yet your Father in heaven takes care of them.
Aren't you worth more than birds?

Matthew 6:26 CEV

BEST YOU CAN

Single moms are doing the best they can. It's not that they can do more or less—they are doing the best they can.

Children with learning disabilities are doing the best they can.

I am doing the best I can.

You are doing the best you can.

Sometimes your best is not enough.
Sometimes it is plenty.

When you do the best you can with what you
have in front of you, it's more than enough
for God—it's pleasing.

Today I choose not to be hard on myself or others. If I had a view from above, I'd see selfless mothers getting their children ready for school and tired parents heading to work. I'd see that people, for the most part, are all just doing the best they can.

Our best makes God smile and that's really all
that should matter. We get caught up on the
thoughts of others, but try and look up! That
smile is the only one that is truly valid, not because
people don't matter, but because as people, we are
all flawed. We are just doing the best we can.

Dear Lord, when I start to beat myself up or am too hard on myself, please remind me where my strength comes from. Lord, I know my best of everything lies with You, so help me choose more of You, so with me, You can do the
BEST YOU CAN.

Let them know that you, whose name is the LORD—that
you alone are the Most High over all the earth.

Psalm 83:18 NIV

MY MOON

Vendy, love is the only thing that lasts forever,
and I am Love

God's great love is like the moon. 🌙 Faithful, forever,
and a witness to all the good in this world.

Vendy, My people are stronger than they think
They are wiser than they think
And they can do more than they think . . . with Me ♡

Dear God, fill me with Your faithful love so I can be all You think.
🌕 My God, establish my faithful steps for the world to see. I, Your
faithful servant, who lives under the moon You created for the world
to see. My forever guide, thank You for the view. May I always
dwell close to You and let Your creation mark my life—acting as a
reminder of how near You are. For as long as the moon is placed in
the sky and the stars shine, my days will belong to You.
Forever will I be Yours, living under
MY MOON.

It will be established forever like the moon, the
faithful witness in the sky.

Psalm 89:37 NIV

OUR DAYS

Our time here is so limited. The days fly by, turning into months, then years pass by before our eyes. Change occurs over the years. Seasons change, people change, and some days I ask myself, "Why? What am I meant to really do with my time?"

The goal is to grow in God's wisdom. Our time here prepares us for eternity with our Creator. Our time here is about growing in His Spirit and taking care of His sheep.

Did you know if a sheep 🐑 is placed on its back, it would be unable to get back upright!

That is us—we are like sheep 🐑 in God's eyes. Not only are we to take care of one another, but our need for our Creator is like that of a baby lamb.

Dear God, because I'm like a sheep and need You to get back up, help me to fill my days with Your wisdom and grow my heart for Your people. 🤍 Lord, I know my days are limited, and although I get mighty impatient with Your plans for me, I know I am like a baby sheep. When life places me on my back, it would be impossible for me to get back up if it weren't for You. So please, I pray with each passing sun, more of Your children learn to invite in Your Spirit to fill OUR DAYS.

Teach us to number our days, that we may gain a heart of wisdom.

Psalm 90:12 NIV

PLENTIFUL

Compassionate: Feeling or showing sympathy
and concern for others.

Gracious: Courteous, kind, and pleasant.

In times of high tension or stress, compassion and kindness can be
hard to find. Where there is God's presence, you will find these two
things. You will find them in the light.

Knowing God's nature brings me peace.
This world may not always be
compassionate, but God is. This world
may not always be kind or pleasant,
but God is.

Dear Lord, grow me during these stressful times. On the busy,
hectic days, share Your overflow of love so there is
plenty for all. Make me
PLENTIFUL.

The Lord is compassionate and gracious, slow to anger, abounding in love.

Psalm 103:8 NIV

GREAT ARE YOU

Lord, great are You. Your creation, Your love, Your promise,
Your glory.

Who is He?
The earth delighted by His work
Satisfied by the produced fruits
He Who waters the mountains from the heavens
He Who plants flowers that give honey and attract bees
He Who directs the sun and moon
Each day, never are they late!

I often find myself confused, not knowing which path to take . . .

Lord, Your foolishness is wiser than
human wisdom and Your weakness
is stronger than human strength.

Dear God, please guide me with Your wisdom. Send her down to
help me! The wisdom that comes from heaven is pure. She helps me
move in peace. She is considerate and helps me see. She is the one
that helps me submit my ways. She is full of mercy and produces
good fruits in me. Impartial and sincere, this wisdom makes me.
That is what I want, and only from You. Please cleanse my heart 🤍
and bless me with this wisdom. Bless all who ask with this wisdom.
All who seek you. 🙏 Oh, great is she, a gift from You, and
GREAT ARE YOU.

He made the moon to mark the seasons, and the sun knows when to go down.
Psalm 104:19 NIV

GATES OF BRONZE AND BARS OF IRON

We all have chains in our lives. Chains of fear, chains of addiction, chains of insecurity, chains of pride—the list goes on and on.

God is full of unfailing love, wonderful deeds, and power unlike any other. His truths have the power to set us free.

God made a way by sending His Son Jesus.
Chains can and will be broken in
His name. Sounds crazy, but it's that
simple. The spilled blood of Jesus
is what makes this true.

God's guiding words—yes, just His words—can
bring you out of darkness. Unlike human words,
God's words are laced with power.

His Scripture is filled with wonderful deeds for mankind, showing us God's nature and empowering people with truth. So I must ask you . . . What gates of bronze and bars of iron do you need God to cut for you?

Dear Lord, there are gates of bronze and bars of iron I have seen You cut through. A people pleaser I was, for twenty-three years I was a slave and "need to please" was my name. But then something happened: I grew really close to You. I read Your words each morning in devotionals and started to hear from You. It was when I started to listen, learn, and lean in that I began to hear more clearly from You. And the truths You gave me are what broke my chains.

So, Father, why don't You do this for more of Your children? I want to hear chains breaking, shattering to the floor due to Your powerful truths! For they are no match for You, these *GATES OF BRONZE AND BARS OF IRON.*

He brought them out of darkness, the utter darkness, and broke away their chains. Let them give thanks to the LORD for his unfailing love and his wonderful deeds for mankind, for he breaks down gates of bronze and cuts through bars of iron.

Psalm 107:14-16 NIV

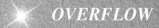 *OVERFLOW*

Generous and just. How do I become this?

I find I can give more on the days I am filled with gratitude. On the days I acknowledge all God has done for my life. I also deeply crave justice for myself and others because I know that is God's heart.
I serve a very just God.

It is easy to do good when there is an overflow. An overflow of love, guidance, protection, wisdom, grace, comfort, and so on.

When we live a life close to God, we can have
peace through uncertainty. We can give more
and take better care of others because we act
and move from a place of overflow.

Dear God, during a time like this, a global pandemic, please take care of all Your people, especially those who are hurting and lacking. May this season teach us compassion, generosity, and justice. May this time tenderize our hearts and cause us to move. Provide for those who need it the most: Your women, children, widows, and orphans! Guide the hearts of Your people, so for all there will be an
OVERFLOW.

Good will come to those who are generous and lend
freely, who conduct their affairs with justice.

Psalm 112:5 NIV

BLESSED BY THE LORD

Flourish: Grow or develop in a healthy or vigorous way, especially as the result of a particularly favorable environment.

What does it look like to flourish by God's standards?

He sets the environment for your life. He fills it with . . .

Healthy, loving, life-giving relationships
Peace of mind
Truth in identity
Safety and nourishment
Rest
Hope
Love

When we flourish with God, everything grows—all areas of our life are affected.

Spending time with my family is always such a blessing for me, but it also opens my eyes to the areas that I do not invite God in enough.

How is it that the people I love the most, I am the least patient with? How is it that the people I love the most (family and friends), I see the least?

Dear God, I do not want to flourish by the ways of this world, demanding a large and empty sacrifice of me. I want to flourish by and with You, the Maker of the heavens and the earth! The blessings from You are much greater. I have given up much time with those I love to chase dreams that this world tells me will fulfill me. I have learned at my ripe age that this is a lie. A huge lie. I am also learning I have no idea what I want, but I know what it will feel like. I might not know what it will look like, but I know what it will feel like. A life filled with love, hope, beauty, truth, kindness, courage, compassion, and rest. I may live in a cute little home by the sea, or on a mountaintop tucked away. I may live in a big, bustling city or in a very isolated place. My dream job might not be what I had thought, nor my lover to be, but that is all okay because I don't know what is best for me, but You do. You are the One Who created me. You are the One Who knows all the things You are able to create with Your hands, greater than my wildest dreams. I think the key is not knowing but trusting. I think the key to unlocking the desires of our hearts is finding delight in You first. Because as long as we don't, we will continue to chase things of this world. Set my heart and mind on fire for You! Today I lay down my old flame to pick up Your new fire, for I am

BLESSED BY THE LORD.

May the LORD cause you to flourish, both you and your children. May you be blessed by the LORD, the Maker of heaven and earth.

Psalm 115:14-15 NIV

WORTHLESS

What is worthless to God?

What do I find worth in?

My understandings are broadened when I try to
comprehend what is important to God.

How do I grow and live a life that preserves the things
of the Lord?

The more I learn about the life of Jesus,
the more unlearning of this world takes
place in me!

Dear God, my ways, thoughts, and desires are so limited. Help
me live a life that follows Your Word for limitless wisdom and
understanding. Preserve my life according to Your Scripture and
teach me of the ways of the Master Teacher Who walked this earth.
Without sin, He defeated the flesh and cravings of the body. He kept
going when He wanted to stop. He chose You when He could have
had anything with a snap of His fingers. He flipped this world upside
down and exposed the king of lies that haunts His people and teases
their eyes with things that are
WORTHLESS.

Turn my eyes away from worthless things,
preserve my life according to your word.

Psalm 119:37 NIV

TIME

God, help me to be grateful for this time, this part of my life, because I know it will never come again. I will never be twenty-four ever again. My family will grow, my grandparents will age, my mom will age, and I will age. The seasons will change, life will change, people will change, and this moment, this day, this time will never be the same.

Yes, You will fill me with joy in new ways,
but some things will never be the same.
Help me appreciate, help me love,
help me enjoy.

I miss the way things used to be, but I know You have far greater days ahead. I miss my family and growing up close to all my loved ones. I miss the simplicity of being sixteen and carefree. I miss the innocent outlook I once had on the world.

Dear God, I know you do not operate in my time, so help me to see You in all things. In the good and the bad, in the waiting and the fulfillment. Help me, lead me, to where you want me. Provide protection for every heart ♥ that seeks to do good and right by You, and send Your Spirit to comfort and lead people everywhere. Please remove the chains of
TIME.

Direct my footsteps according to your
word; let no sin rule over me.

Psalm 119:133 NIV

☀ *LAMP FOR MY FEET* ☀

I constantly take my life into my own hands . . .

I constantly pray and don't believe . . .

But my heart 🤍 is set on keeping Your ways to the very end. You always give me discernment and understanding, so I can have a view from above.

🔑 Great peace He gives to those who crave His will. His laws make it so nothing, not even death, can make us fall. 😌

Dear God, thank You for all the moments in my life spent alone with You. I wish to load my life with more of these moments. These moments with You fill me, give me peace, understanding, and comfort. I pray all Your people get to experience more of You, Your ways, and Your moves. You are the only thing that will not fail us. 🙏 You are a
LAMP FOR MY FEET!

Your word is a lamp for my feet, a light on my path.

Psalm 119:105 NIV

REST

Some nights I sleep better than others. Some days I rest more than others. When I trust God, I find rest—regardless of my workload, worries, or fears.

The world is slowing down right now. Some people are finding rest and being restored while others are restless, full of worry and fear.

Only your Creator can grant you
true rest. Accept it, don't fight it.
He always has a plan for those who
ASK and **SEEK**.

When you work for God, He will
give you rest.

Dear God, if it's not from You, then I don't want it to be blessed. Your will and Your will only, Lord. No more early mornings or late nights unless they are for You! For too long I have done things in my own strength. It is not until Your children learn to be still that they find true
REST.

In vain you rise early, and stay up late, toiling for
food to eat—for he grants sleep to those he loves.

Psalm 127:2 NIV

SUN AND MOON

God created the sun to rise every morning and the moon for the
nights. How beautiful and perfect this is.

Vendy, when the sun rises each morning,
know how loved you are
Vendy, when the moon rises each night,
know how loved you are

His love is made to endure forever.

Dear Lord, I pray more of Your children grow to know Your love.
If more of us were reminded of Your constant and never-ending
love, if more of us knew and felt this love, we would choose things
that bring us peace and not harm. Love changes the way people see
themselves, and as a result, it changes their choices. God, may the
risings and settings act as reminders of Your enduring love.
Each day may we look to the
SUN AND MOON.

The sun to govern the day, His love endures forever. The moon
and stars to govern the night; His love endures forever.

Psalm 136:8-9 NIV

APRIL

DOUBT

God never gives us a spirit of doubt or confusion, but there will be times in our lives where we have to choose, and doubt is knocking at the door. How do we know when we are walking in His will or making the right decision?

Prayer. Pour out every concern at His feet.

Trust that it truly is in His hands and there is nothing more you can do.

God, if I trust You . . . truly and fully, I can let go and know You will make it right. You will make my path straight. Please help me to fully trust and surrender it to You.

Dear Lord, please help me to trust **YOU**. Not my circumstances, not my actions, not my feelings, not people, not all I see, not all I feel, but **YOU**. My God, I cry to You and pour out my heart to You with the things that trouble me because they become too much! So today I need Your help fighting the doubt before I make a decision that is not of Your true and beautiful will. Or even worse, does not honor You, the One Who has always done right by me . . . I just can't let this be! Please, Father, speak to me, show me what I need to see and remove my

DOUBT.

I cry aloud to the LORD; I lift up my voice to the LORD for mercy. I pour out before him my complaint; before him I tell my trouble. When my spirit grows faint within me, it is you who watch over my way.

Psalm 142:1-3 NIV

YOUR WILL

Teach: To show or explain how to do something.

Lead: Cause (a person or animal) to go with one
by holding them by the hand, while moving forward.
To be a route or means of access to a particular place
or in a particular direction.

Through His unfailing love, we are able to
walk on level ground.

Dear God, show and explain Your will to me. Hold my hand and
move me on the route of Your choice. My loving God, You are my
light, my protection against every fear, anxious thought, and painful
experience. Thank You for all Your love. Please help me hand my
life over to You each and every day. Father, I crave
YOUR WILL.

Teach me to do your will, for you are my God;
may your good Spirit lead me on level ground.

Psalm 143:10 NIV

RICH LOVE

Your goodness is never-ending. Your goodness never fails. Your heart 🤍 is what I crave. Your compassion, rich love, and gentle spirit give me rest. Oh, You are so good to me, You Who created me!

God opens our blind eyes to the joy found in the simplicity of His creation. He helps us live close to Him in a world that is far from Him and His ways.

Dear Lord, thank You for all You have done. I pray this world 🌍 gets to experience You in fullness. In all Your wonder, in all Your glory. God, I pray to be more like You . . . gracious and compassionate, slow to anger, and forgiving. I need help though, my flesh at times gets the best of me; so grow my heart, grow it in *RICH LOVE.*

The LORD is gracious and compassionate, slow to anger and rich in love. The LORD is good to all; he has compassion on all he has made.

Psalm 145:8-9 NIV

RISE AGAIN

Vendy, I just want My creation to enjoy the blessings
and the fruits of their lives I made possible

Because of You, Jesus, my life is filled with so much beauty. It is
all around me. It is everywhere I look, my dear God. You are my
light. My comfort and my peace. I will never fully understand
Your goodness or this world, but thank You for defeating death and
making a way.

Your love lives in the hearts and minds of people everywhere. Death
could not silence what has been freely given.

Nothing can undo what He has already done. Because
He rose from the dead, you will rise again!

Dear Jesus, I had hope when I shouldn't have had hope. I had peace
when I shouldn't have had peace. I overcame when much was
against me. I was able to do this because of what You have done.
Thank You. My God, You made a way when there was no way. I
want to give my life to You today because I owe You my everything.
I have never experienced such darkness, but I no longer fear the
night, Lord, because of what Your innocent body strung to a cross
did. I do not fully understand why God chose to send You as a
Savior for the world . . . but I also do not fully understand God and
why He does much of what He does because His ways are so much
higher than mine. But I write all of this to testify to this truth—

because of You, people all around the world who face circumstances
and battles much greater than themselves will learn to
RISE AGAIN.

For this God is our God for ever and ever;
he will be our guide even to the end.

Psalm 48:14 NIV

KEYS FROM HEAVEN

I GIVE

Wisdom: The quality of having experience, knowledge, and good judgment.

Knowledge: Facts, information, and skills acquired by a person through experience or education.

Understanding: Sympathetically aware of other people's feelings; tolerant and forgiving.

God gives insight as if you experienced it.

Dear God, almost always, when I don't know what to do so much so that it pains me, I am very good at running to You. This is a skill set I have cultivated that was not always there, but the point is, from You comes wisdom, knowledge, and understanding that outweighs any input from a human being because You are the beginning and the end. You know what will happen before it even happens. You know all things. You are the Creator of all, so what is it You cannot give? You fill me with wisdom and make it so

I GIVE.

For the LORD gives wisdom; from his mouth come
knowledge and understanding.

Proverbs 2:6 NIV

TABLET OF YOUR HEART

Wisdom brings peace and prosperity.

Peace = freedom from disturbance
Prosperity = flourishing, success in all forms

How do we gain more wisdom?

We pray and ask God for more of her.

We meditate on God's Word.

We listen to her ways, keep His teachings in our
heart , and she will bestow well-being.

Wisdom is a gift from God. Wisdom is not our own
understanding, but the ways of our Creator.

Dear Lord, wisdom and I have grown close these past few years.
She has taught me many things. She has taught me to say less and
listen more. To be still and wait on You before I move. To lead with
kindness always so I will never have regrets. She has taught me the
beauty and power in simplicity. Long walks, time in Your creation,
and much reflection. She has clothed me in beauty and laced my
steps with honor and faithfulness. She is steadfast and not quick to
change her mind, but slow and steady. She guides with divine

power and creates kings out of fools! She is the way to victory because she is of and from You. She is Your creation and those who seek will receive. Those who bend a knee get her along with all of the fruits she produces. She makes it so one cannot go wrong in this crooked world in Your sight. She has transformed me, and I know she is special because her ways are all written on the
TABLET OF YOUR HEART.

Let love and faithfulness never leave you; bind them around your neck, write them on the tablet of your heart. Then you will win favor and a good name in the sight of God and man.

Proverbs 3:3-4 NIV

WISDOM CALLS

Why do we as humans need wisdom?

If we don't need it, why is it good for us?

Wisdom brings the quality of being well. When we
make wise decisions, our hearts and minds
are protected and our mental health thrives.

What good is it to have everything and more with no
peace of mind?

What is quality of life without a sound mind? No
sound mind, no ability to enjoy.

God's wisdom = protection for every step you take.

Dear God, none of our desires compare to the beauty of wisdom.
She is all-knowing and a gift 📖 from You. I pray for wisdom in all
Your people so their minds and hearts will be protected by You. 🙏
So good in this world will be done and people will have peace in
all areas. Everyone, she is ready to give freely. Seek Him, men and
women, and you will find her, for
WISDOM CALLS!

For wisdom is more precious than rubies, and
nothing you desire can compare with her.

Proverbs 8:11 NIV

HELP ME TO LOVE

How do we honestly love when someone upsets us?
When someone hurts us or the people we care about?

Love is a choice, not a feeling.

Even if you don't feel love for someone, in the midst of how you feel, you can still choose to treat them with love and respect. I struggle so much with this, and a very dear friend, also my roomie, reminds me, "Vendela, your feelings will catch up . . . lead with love."

How easy is it to love those who love you?

Dear God, help me to love not just those who are good and kind to me, but those who need it the most. Those who are lost, confused, and who hurt others. Father, when I am dealing with these people, give me the words—not the words stirred by my feelings, but the words that are smooth like honey to calm the conflict. Father, help me love because it covers all wrongs and makes it so I can truly forgive. Father, when I love, it is You Who dwells in me. So even if I interact with souls who do not know the Son but know love, they have You, the mighty Creator, in them because You are Love.
So please, Father,
HELP ME TO LOVE.

Hatred stirs up conflict, but love
covers over all wrongs.

Proverbs 10:12 NIV

HUMILITY

When I see someone I admire do great things with humility, it makes me want to be humble.

When I am told by someone I care about to be humble,
I then want to be humble.

When I get praised for something God whispered in my ear or brought me through, I am humbled.

Pride is full of lies, and pride rips you
away from what you love.

Dear God, help me to be humble. Humility is sweet, beautiful, and smooth as honey. 😊 It drips with love and honor and points to You. Help me to always know where my river of life stems from. Father, when I think of the most humble human being, I think of Your Son. The One Who walked this earth, commanded the wind to stop, and raised the dead back to life. I think of He Who could do all things, but remained silent and oftentimes meek. He was never fearful or timid, but when dealing with others He moved with love and gentleness. He cared for the lost with kindness and compassion and helped all who were in need. Father, clothe me in this, teach me more of Jesus'
HUMILITY.

When pride comes, then comes disgrace, but with humility comes wisdom.

Proverbs 11:2 NIV

PRODUCING ABUNDANCE

Generosity = Prosperity

When we are generous with people, with our wealth, with what we have, we will prosper in all forms—love, hope, faith, and so on.

Whoever refreshes others will
be refreshed.

We are living in a season where there is a sense of lack and fear. About 3.3 million people in the United States alone just lost their jobs. How do we combat?

Move forward free from fear.

When we are fearful, we do not give because we believe there will not be enough. God blesses generosity in all forms. Now is a time to give fearlessly.

Dear Lord, I do not know if I am one to speak on giving, as You have provided and always blessed me. But as I grew and ventured out on my own, away from the protection and love of my family, I have seen the ways people treat others cheaply. The hurtful measures of corporations who treat people with families as numbers on their excel sheets. Yes, this has always hurt me, but rather than letting it get the best of me, I was encouraged to be the change. Do it differently. So when I deal with others, I will never let this be.

And Father, if I do . . . well, then speak to the fear that is dictating me because I never want to not give, not refresh, especially when You have always been so generous to me! Lord, You make us prosper beyond belief,
PRODUCING ABUNDANCE.

One person gives freely, yet gains even more; another withholds unduly, but comes to poverty. A generous person will prosper; whoever refreshes others will be refreshed.

Proverbs 11:24-25 NIV

GREAT UNDERSTANDING

Patient = Understanding

I lack much understanding at times, which is why I ask God to help me be patient. Patient so He can show me what I am missing, all I don't see.

Patient: Able to accept or tolerate delays, problems, or suffering without becoming annoyed or anxious.

I believe when one is patient, they are confident.
They know what is supposed to happen for them
will—maybe not exactly on their timeline, but
only in a matter of time.

Dear God, please help me to be patient with my family, friends, and those I care about. Help me to be patient for Your will and the desires of my heart. Help me to gain great understanding so I can stay on Your path. With patience, Lord, comes no regrets. With patience, Father, comes fruits and blessings beyond our wildest dreams. Lord, as I remain patient, bring joy to me. Bring joy to Your children, the ones that learn to wait on You and Your time. Please, Lord, honor them. My God, with all these gifts come great responsibility and stewardship You give us. Lord, please continue to grant Your people
GREAT UNDERSTANDING.

Whoever is patient has great understanding, but
one who is quick-tempered displays folly.

Proverbs 14:29 NIV

HUMAN HEART

In the beginning, God knew the course of our lives. He knew where we would be born. He knew all our firsts. He knows all our lasts.

Why then, if we have an all-knowing and powerful God, do our human hearts, our human minds, take matters into our own hands? Why, when I have an all-knowing God, do I do this time and time again?

The spirit indeed is willing, but the flesh is weak. With these two against each other, we **MUST** pray for His will to be done. I pray for God's will to be done in my life, the lives of all those I love, and all those who desire God's truth.

God, You have placed beautiful, wonderful plans on my heart and my human self has a way of twisting them . . . putting pressure and a timeline on things that I could have never even dreamed of without You, let alone accomplished.

Dear Lord, direct each and every one of my steps. Purify my heart so Your blessings do not become gods and plans do not consume me. Please, Lord, keep my intentions and will pure. Lord, direct my every step and strengthen my
HUMAN HEART.

In their hearts humans plan their course, but the Lord establishes their steps.

Proverbs 16:9 NIV

FOOD FOR THE SOUL

What is sweet for our souls?

What is healing to our bones?

Kind and considerate words.

They go a long way for a friend who needs encouragement, for a parent who is hard on themselves, for a coworker who is stressed, and for yourself.

Kind and considerate words can cause breakthroughs and realizations amid confusion, anger, and hate.

Kind and considerate words are sweet. They put out fires. They are laced with truth and can help deep wounds to heal.

When God gives wisdom, your lips
promote instruction. Instruction
sweet as honey 🍯 and healing to all.

Dear Lord, kindness has indeed brought healing to my soul. It's the kindness I have experienced when I least expected it or needed it the most. I almost think of those kind words as divine interventions. It's not that the kind words were the most profound thing, but the timing. The kind words delivered just when you need it the most—now that is powerful. Kindness, I do believe, is divine and from You. It is something You delight in, so there must be power in this! Kindness

and compassion from another human soul on my busiest most stressed days has kept me going. Lord, I pray more of Your people spread this beautiful thing because it is truly
FOOD FOR THE SOUL.

Gracious words are a honeycomb, sweet
to the soul and healing to the bones.

Proverbs 16:24 NIV

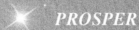

PROSPER

Truth in wisdom∽life full of joy∽understanding
births perspective∽a prosperous life is filled with peace

Get wisdom and you will love your life.

Cherish understanding and you
will soon prosper.

A prosperous life is available to all
who ask and seek. 🤍

Dear Lord, in time we will prosper. First must come the
understanding of You and Your ways, then come Your friends
wisdom and self-control! And at last comes the blessings that cause
us to fly high into the sky. Above the pain, shame, loss, and hurt . . .
above it all. Father, I am ready to love my life! I have been down for
some time, but in a hidden place growing my wings and training in
wisdom, compassion, and understanding. Now it is time, my Lord.
Show me what it looks like to
PROSPER!

The one who gets wisdom loves life; the one who
cherishes understanding will soon prosper.

Proverbs 19:8 NIV

SECURITY

People steal from the innocent; hardworking people lose their jobs; sickness strikes the pure; and people who tell the truth get punished for it.

Does this world truly offer security . . . ?

🗝 Through love, you are protected.
Protected from fear, protected
from hate, protected from evil.

🗝 Some places need more love. 🤍

Dear God, I pray for more love, not just in families and homes 🏠 but in the working world, in corporations, in prisons and mental hospitals, in places that need it most. I pray for more love—love that produces faith, kindness, courage, and wisdom—so the lives of others will be put first. I pray people win the battle over fear. May Your light win. May the kings and queens of this world make decisions out of love, creating security for humanity. I pray in Jesus' name 🙏 for Your people to experience this *SECURITY.*

Love and faithfulness keep a king safe; through
love his throne is made secure.

Proverbs 20:28 NIV

FRIENDSHIP WITH A KING

What would it be like to be friends with the king?

You'd have certain access, privilege (special rights, advantages, or immunities), possible power and authority over matters that are close to your heart, access to great meals 😂, and insights on rulings, maybe?

To be close friends with a king gives behind-the-scenes knowledge and information. You know the operations of his authority. Since you are friends, you want him to win. You know how good his heart is, the protection he provides, so you want his will to be done.

When we are friends with Jesus, these are just some of the benefits that stem from that relationship.

Jesus is King. There is power in just His name, and there are benefits to having Him as a friend.

Dear Lord, help me to love with a pure heart and speak truth with grace. May Your rule reign in my heart and the hearts of others everywhere so they live in Your peaceful kingdom of plenty. 🙏 Lord, please bless me with *FRIENDSHIP WITH A KING.*

One who loves a pure heart and who speaks with grace will have the king for a friend.

Proverbs 22:11 NIV

REFRESHED SPIRIT

God, You act as my messenger. You grant me encouragement and comfort when I need it most. You offer full and complete love. When I am hard on myself, You shine a light in the darkness.

You are God, so You can always do this, but so can we—for others—if we are honest and trustworthy.

A friend who is truthful is a friend you never want to lose. A person with a pure heart that speaks truth is a light for your steps. A guide when you need it most. What could be more valuable than this?

When you are honest and truthful with people, they grow in respect for you. Not because they always agree with what you have to say, or even like what you have to say, but because they know your words stem from a pure place. Truth sets people free.

The truth is not always easy to speak, but it will always honor what is right.

Dear Lord, a key from heaven is like a bridge that leads one to the divine. Please help me wait on You for these truths! Help me wait on You for these keys to fall, for they come when I sit and am still with You. Your keys drench me in truth, providing me with a *REFRESHED SPIRIT.*

Like a snow-cooled drink at harvest time is a trustworthy messenger
to the one who sends him; he refreshes the spirit of his master.

Proverbs 25:13 NIV

UNSTOPPABLE

Jesus, Your Spirit makes us unstoppable.

We can go through anything and come out on the other side with a smile on our faces. You can give us joy and peace in the midst of a storm. You can do the **IMPOSSIBLE** in our lives because nothing is impossible for You.

I woke up this morning feeling very grateful. Grateful to see another day. Grateful to sit and reflect. Grateful for all the good that's happened thus far in my life. Grateful for all the bad that You have brought me through.

Jesus, if I didn't have Your Spirit, I wouldn't be happy. I wouldn't see the world through Your lens, and I wouldn't rise up with gratitude today.

Lord, may You do work in our lives that only You can do. May our lives reflect Your heart. 🤍 May Your creation rise up and be unstoppable through You.

Dear God, I am thankful for You, the things You say, the things You hear, and the things You tell me! My special messenger. I pray You encourage and empower Your people today. I pray they feel the warm light Your love gives off, and I pray for comfort in the hearts and minds of people everywhere. No matter what we lose or gain, we will never be able to lose Your eternal love for us and the life that stems from that love. Thank You for making us *UNSTOPPABLE*.

As water reflects the face, so one's life reflects the heart.
Proverbs 27:19 NIV

BLANKETS

God, I don't understand Your goodness, but I know
Your love.

God's love is vast, never-ending, and always there when
You need it. God's love is truthful, and His love will be
a bright light that keeps you moving forward and keeps
you from getting lost.

I love all My creation,
but I am close to the brokenhearted
I wrap My love around them like a blanket,
so they know Me
My people have hearts and minds
that hear from Me and crave Me
Because they have tasted My goodness
If you live long enough, My goodness
makes no sense in this world
But that's also what makes it so powerful
I send blankets down from heaven
And the sweet taste of kindness is a byproduct of the
warmth provided by My blankets

Dear Lord, I pray for many more blankets, many more tender hearts,
and many more cares . . . leading us to many more dreams.
Wrap us in Your love and send down Your
BLANKETS.

A dream comes when there are many cares.

Ecclesiastes 5:3 NIV

MAY

MUCH MORE

We learn, we learn, we learn.

What use is pain? I've run from it, avoided it all my life in every way I could until something knocked me down and I had no choice but to face it.

We learn, we learn, we learn.

Pain births sorrow and grief. And when embraced and welcomed with God by your side, you can and will walk through that pain and come out on the other side with more wisdom, more knowledge, and more strength.

I don't know why that's the formula, but it just is. So, Lord, I just ask, please don't ever let me suffer without You. I don't ever want to know a world without You.

Dear God, I pray we are able to see the beauty in every season and situation of life, no matter how heavy or grief-filled it is. For this is something that only You can gift and do. Bless us with joy in the midst of great pain and turn our weakness into our strength. For with You, there is always
MUCH MORE.

For with much wisdom comes much sorrow;
the more knowledge, the more grief.

Ecclesiastes 1:18 NIV

MY GOODNESS

I see the trees bend with the gentle breeze, I see golden light shine down from the sky and kiss the earth. I see lush greenery, with pops of color poking out. I smell the ocean, hear the sea, I feel the warmth of the sun, and I'm grateful for my time here. Alone. Just with You. Just breathing. Just being. Able to feel whatever I need to feel.

I do not deserve Your goodness, but I'm so grateful. 🤍
I don't want to leave this time. This time, this moment in time where I feel so at peace. Where I feel so very at peace.

Let Me, your God, give you rest
Let Me, your Lord, give you joy
Let me, your God, give you everything
and don't question My goodness
Just enjoy

It is always a good time to embrace His goodness.

Dear Lord, I don't like the hurry. I don't like the rush. I don't like the pressure. I don't like the what-ifs. I just want to sit and be with You. Thank You, Lord, for today. Thank You for the time we have together. I pray to learn from this season, to create stronger boundaries that hold and protect our time. I pray for the peace of this rest to follow Your people back into the ordinary. I pray for this time to be part of our everyday grind. Our everyday walk. Our everyday being. May this time follow me throughout my day. Oh, it is what I crave, it is what I need. May our time always be what makes the way. Oh, how this time scatters

MY GOODNESS.

A time to scatter stones and a time to gather them, a time to embrace and a time to refrain from embracing.

Ecclesiastes 3:5 NIV

ENDURE FOREVER

What do we have that will endure forever?

Our jobs will not.
Our houses will not.
Our lives will not.

The only thing we, as humans, can do that
will endure forever is love.

Spread love and kindness to people. It lives in their hearts, gets
passed down from generation to generation, friendship to friendship,
family member to family member, and becomes a
part of our souls when we enter heaven.

Love shapes us as humans.

God is Love, so when we love, we endure
forever with Him.

Dear Lord, You do not give us a spirit of fear, but if we truly knew
Your power, we would fear You because there is nothing You cannot
do. Please help me to fear You and cultivate Your love so the days
of my life are not wasted by toil under the sun, but filled with hope,
faith, love, and Your Spirit that allows my soul to
ENDURE FOREVER.

I know that everything God does will endure forever; nothing
can be added to it and nothing taken from it. God does it so that
people will fear him.

Ecclesiastes 3:14 NIV

VERY FEW

God is in heaven. Heaven is not part of earth. Heaven is above. God is omnipotent and omniscient.

If God tells me not to be quick with my mouth and less is more with my words, then there must be power in His silence that I do not understand.

When we are wise, we are blameless. We don't give reason for others to come against our character or word—though they may try.

When our words are few, there is less to come against. When our words are few, God can move and speak in the silence. He whispers in people's hearts and minds.

God will step in and make all things right on behalf of the blameless.

Dear Lord, help me to be less concerned with my stance, for I know You are my foundation and provider . . . because of this I will always be in good hands. Nothing is more powerful than You. God, help me to be more concerned with the needs of others. So I don't waste my few words and they are used only where You'd like them to be. It is Your view from above that gets me through. Your view

makes me as wise as a serpent and as gentle as a dove as I move
about in the midst of evil, pushing Your agenda to the forefront!
Your whispers direct my steps in this game of chess and
keep my words
VERY FEW.

Do not be quick with your mouth, do not be hasty in your heart to utter
anything before God. God is in heaven and you are on earth, so let your
words be few.

Ecclesiastes 5:2 NIV

SEE THE SUN

What would this world look like if there was no sun?

We would stumble for sure; with the help of electricity, we could manage, but where there is no light, we would definitely fall. Maybe we'd suffer from a lack of vitamin D and our beautiful plants would not make it!

Wisdom is like the sun. Bright and beautiful, it provides warmth and fuel for your body and soul. Without it, we would stumble.

Dear God, You are full of wisdom. Wisdom is a gift from You. She is kind to everyone and benefits those who seek her ways. Lord, please send down more wisdom so we can have more vitamin D for our souls, so we can walk with a light as our guide for each step and look up to
SEE THE SUN.

Wisdom, like an inheritance, is a good thing
and benefits those who see the sun.

Ecclesiastes 7:11 NIV

WHAT IF

We will all die. No one knows the exact span of their life, or how long they will be here, but they do know that at one point they will die because death happens to all of us. Some die young, some die old, some in between.

So when times are good, be happy.

That may just be for a day, an hour, a moment, or a feeling. But whatever it is, enjoy it. Soak it up. Soak it in. Because times will not always be good, and times will not always be bad. There are seasons in life. There are waves in life.

Today was a good day and I am grateful. For the clean food I put in my body, for the sun on my skin, for the air in my lungs, for the love that surrounds me, for the peace of today. The stress-free nature of today. The excitement of today. The purity of today. I may not always have days like today, so, God, I want to be happy and alive to the goodness of today.

The timeline of my life is something only You know. I may fill my mind with useless thoughts, and painful what-ifs. What if I lose another person I love? What if I could do more? What if I could be better? What if I . . .

Dear Lord, death does not scare me. I look forward to one day being fully with You. But a life full of what if, could have, should have, does scare me. A life full of wanting to love more but holding back does scare me. I pray my family knows and feels my love. I pray my friends know and feel my love. I pray for a life of happiness when times are good. I pray, Father, against the

"WHAT IF."

As no one has power over the wind to contain it, so
no one has power over the time of their death.

Ecclesiastes 8:8 NIV

WORK OF GOD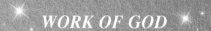

I do not understand You. I do not understand why You allow certain things to happen and don't allow others. I do not understand Your goodness. I do not understand how vast Your heart is. I do not know why You have blessed me. Blessed me with so much. So much that I fail to see, that I fail to enjoy. But that's Your goodness.

I do not understand Your timeline, but it's all I want. You, the Maker of all things. I want to enjoy my life with You. I want to enjoy all that's from You because it may not be here tomorrow. Because it may never come again.

Dear Lord, thank You for today. Thank You for the sweet memories of my life, my childhood, and everything leading to today. The simplicity of it all. I love You. 🖤 You are the Maker of all that is good. I pray my life reflects the *WORK OF GOD.*

As you do not know the path of the wind, or how the body is formed in a mother's womb, so you cannot understand the work of God, the Maker of all things.

Ecclesiastes 11:5 NIV

ALWAYS HERE

Thank You, Lord, for always being near. When I'm sad, You are near to me. When I'm happy, You are near to me. My dear Lord, thank You.

Some days my little heart 🤍 hurts or feels heavy, and I don't always know why. I try to remind myself of all I should be grateful for, but even then, my mind wanders!

Be still. He will put you at ease, comfort you, and strengthen you beyond belief.

He fights the fear. He fights the heaviness.

Dear God, I feel most comforted in silence and stillness with You. This is something I can always go back to. Thank You for stillness. Thank you for the quiet. Thank you, Lord. Oh, I love You and how You are always near and
ALWAYS HERE.

The Lord will fight for you; you need only to be still.

Exodus 14:14 NIV

FAITH

What is faith? Believing without seeing.

Faith is the assurance that the things revealed and promised in God's Word are true, even though unseen.

To stand? Two feet planted, best when on a firm surface.

What does it look like to stand firm in your faith?

To trust with your heart and mind.

It's easy for me to trust in my heart, but I find it hard to trust with my mind. To place God's promises and words before my own thoughts. To place weight in His promises and live with them each day.

Faith gives a believer conviction that what he expects in faith will come to pass. It becomes so tangible that you now possess it. It becomes a reality.

Dear Lord, me of little faith . . . I really need Your help believing many of the things You have promised and spoken to me because many of them, I cannot see. Many of them will happen in Your time, many of them appear to be impossible, and many of them take mighty **FAITH!** Grow Your believers in faith. And those who don't believe in You . . . speak to their hearts because it is You Who created them, and You Who loves them. Father, You speak to my heart first, then I battle my thoughts and force them to bend a knee to You. I constantly have to meet lies with truth. Your truth fights the lies that combat Your words. Father, may Your people win the battle of the mind and stand firm in their

FAITH.

If you do not stand firm in your faith, you will not stand at all.

Isaiah 7:9 NIV

STRENGTH OF MY HAND

The power in just His hand. Bad things will happen, but by the strength of His hand, He makes those bad things bow to Him.

We are living in a time where nations and people are realizing what little value is in the things of this world. Worldly treasures mean nothing if you can't leave your home.

God is wise, and there is nothing that can overpower Him or His hand. There is nothing that is too stressful, great, or challenging for Him. He created all things.

Only God can silence the world and the rulers of this world. Only God can expose false gods because there is nothing He cannot do.

He is good, He is faithful, and His hand makes all things in the world right. If we can just use this time to be strengthened by His hand, what will we look like? What will this world look like?

Dear God, You will remove the boundaries of nations, plunder their treasures, and subdue their kings should it be Your will. Your Spirit is up to something oh so mighty in my life because I fell in love, deep love with You first. And this love is what keeps me going, directs my steps, and what will subdue kings. I just pray that Your will be done on earth as it is in heaven by the strength of Your hand, and not by the
STRENGTH OF MY HAND.

For he says: "By the strength of my hand I have done this, and by my wisdom, because I have understanding. I removed the boundaries of nations, I plundered their treasures; like a mighty one I subdued their kings."

Isaiah 10:13 NIV

MORE THAN ENOUGH

Vendy, you can be alone
You can have nothing but Me
and still have more than enough

How?

I created all things,
all that is true and beautiful comes from Me
I am more than the things I created

The things you miss some days—family and friends, a love, a dream—God created all those things. He planted the dream and blessed you with the relationships. They all give color to life, but without them, He is still more than enough.

Dear God, I thank You for another day on earth 🌍 , not because it was the best day, but because with You I have more than enough. With You everything else is sprinkled on top. I pray more of Your believers and people reach this point in their faith. I pray they know and believe in their hearts that because of Jesus, You, Father, will meet all our needs, and with You we will always have *MORE THAN ENOUGH.*

And my God will meet all your needs according
to the riches of his glory in Christ Jesus.

Philippians 4:19 NIV

YOKE OF THE WORLD

A time to rain
A time for sun
A time for sleep
A time to run

With You, Lord, the yoke is light. Help me to see this. Help me to believe this. My feelings of worry and fear are not welcome. Not today, tomorrow, or any day. With You the weight is light. The load is light. My steps are light.

Ask God to open your eyes to the
blessings, to all He does.

Dear Lord, when things do not go as I have planned and hoped for, my mind is robbed of its peace. But because, Father, I gave my life to You and I desire to choose You, I know the plan of the Lord Almighty will be done with me. You have determined a plan for the whole world, not just me. This plan is stretched over all nations and is for thousands of generations. Who can thwart the hand of God? Who is more powerful than You? Take my yoke today and send reminders of this. With You there is a time for everything, a time for everything under the sun. In Your hand is the
YOKE OF THE WORLD.

This is the plan determined for the whole world; this is the hand stretched out
over all nations. For the LORD Almighty has purposed, and who can thwart
him? His hand is stretched out, and who can turn it back?

Isaiah 14:26-27 NIV

NEW CREATION

Your love is more vast than the ocean.

When water is released, it knows no boundaries. There is no hole You do not fill when Your love is released.

Healing: Alleviate, correct, and make right.

Your love brings healing.

Your love is enough. Your love alleviates pain and suffering in our lives. It corrects and makes new.

Dear Lord, I pray for the old to be gone and the new to come by the power of Christ Jesus and Your love! I pray for healing of the minds, souls, and bodies of those who suffer everywhere. All those who suffer mentally and physically. All the brokenhearted, Father. For if they do not experience love in the midst of their suffering, they may turn to things that bring them more harm, more hurt, more pain, and more shame. I know this because when I was the most broken after my loss, I was the most tempted to turn to more hurt and pain because that was all I could feel. I know this can happen because it has happened to my sister. I have seen it happen to those I love firsthand. God, if anyone accepts Your Son and invites Him into their pain, the old will be gone. In the old is the pain and shame, the lies and hurts, that stop the new. I pray for more souls to be renewed by You. May this world be filled with more people who are new, a *NEW CREATION.*

Therefore, if anyone is in Christ, the new creation
has come: The old has gone, the new is here!

2 Corinthians 5:17 NIV

PLANNED LONG AGO

God is perfect. He does wonderful things, things that were planned long ago.

Perfect faithfulness: What He says
will come to be.

Wonderful things: Any and everything
good in your life.

Dear Lord, thank You for another beautiful day. The sunshine is from You, the peace of an early morning is from You. The singing birds are from You. A loving parent is from You. An encouraging friend is from You. I pray to lead my life with Your joy. Stress removed. Anxiousness removed. Expectations removed. Just peace from Your love and light above for, Father, You have things in store for me—for us all, I know—that You
PLANNED LONG AGO.

LORD, you are my God; I will exalt you and praise your name,
for in perfect faithfulness you have done wonderful things,
things planned long ago.

Isaiah 25:1 NIV

FRAGILE HEART

That's what I do to My people, Vendy,
I make them highly sensitive and aware
I make their hearts and minds tender
and pure for the goodness of others

A fragile heart is a tender heart. When something
is tender, it's cooked perfectly. Not overcooked,
not undercooked. It's just right.

I make your heart just right
Just right for heaven
If you feel overwhelmed,
it's because tender hearts on earth
are mixed and spread wide
They are mixed with overcooked hearts
and undercooked hearts

Invite God to have control over your heart.

Let Me control your heart
I will give you wisdom, grace, and peace
to live full and abundantly with a tender heart
One that knows how to thrive
on earth and heaven

Dear Lord, I want to wait for You. I am a fragile heart living in
a world far from You. I see things that pain me; they hurt my heart.
I see things that bring me to my knees and cause me to pray to You.
I see things that cause me to turn to You and walk in Your ways and
keep Your laws—not always because I want to. You have cooked
my heart, Lord, made it just right. My spirit longs for You.
Lord, take care of us, watch over and protect the people in
this world who have a
FRAGILE HEART.

Yes, LORD, walking in the way of your laws, we wait for you; your name
and renown are the desire of our hearts. My soul yearns for you in the
night; in the morning my spirit longs for you.

Isaiah 26:8-9 NIV

FRUITFUL VINEYARD

I am from the Napa Valley. I grew up with vineyards, and vineyards are beautiful. Rolling hills of greenery with bright, plump, purple treats hanging from their branches. Large green leaves provide shade from the sun that shines down. Vineyards are lovely. They produce and provide fruits.

God will guard you day and night. He will grow your vineyard, tend to your fields, watch over you continually, and guard you day and night so no harm may ever come to your vineyard.

Dear God, You have guarded my heart and mind for twenty-five years and one day today. You have watered me and never stopped. You have opened my eyes to Your goodness. I hope to spend the next twenty-five years singing about Your fruitful vineyards all over the world. Father, may more souls invite You into their lives. May more souls partner with You to produce a *FRUITFUL VINEYARD.*

Sing about a fruitful vineyard: I, the LORD, watch over it;
I water it continually. I guard it day and night so that no
one may harm it.

Isaiah 27:2-3 NIV

TEACHINGS AND INSTRUCTIONS

Lord, Your way is the only way I want. Not because
I understand, not because it's comfortable, but because I know it's
magnificent. It's wonderful and greater than anything my mind can
think of or create.

His plan is wonderful.

His wisdom is magnificent.

Dear God, You planted in me desires and dreams. Help me hand
them over to You so they follow Your timeline and divine plan.
These plans are wonderful, and I need Your magnificent wisdom to
navigate them. Father, give me the roadmap and the keys to
the vehicle of Your choice, then write on my heart Your
TEACHINGS AND INSTRUCTIONS.

All this also comes from the LORD Almighty, whose
plan is wonderful, whose wisdom is magnificent.

Isaiah 28:29 NIV

DWELL

When I think of peace, I think of my mind.
Peace of mind. When I think of a peaceful dwelling,
I imagine no stress. When I think of safety, I imagine
the comfort of my home.

Peace: Completeness, success, fulfillment, wholeness, harmony,
security, and well-being.

Dwell: Formal, literary to live as a permanent
resident, to live.

Safety: Freedom from danger or hazard.

God grants us peaceful dwelling and safety at all
times from this world.

When we have this, when we believe His words and they become
part of us, very few things scare us because we know when God
creates a dwelling place in our life, we are protected from all harm
and gifted peace.

Things will happen that you have no control over—strange things,
challenging things—but with God as your dwelling place, you have
full and complete peace. I just know this to be true because of
what I walked through. I do not fully understand how He does it,
but I know He does.

Dear God, You have allowed my stressed, hurt, and broken heart to lie down and sleep. You created a safe dwelling for me. You did what no human could do. Father, please do this for others. For the women, the children, the good men, and those who live far from You. Father, I know Your favor is on me, but maybe You can place Your favor on others too? Share the light, the love, and the peace that stems from only You? I have accepted Jesus because of Your love for me, so maybe that's the key? For those to do the same? If so, Father, then I pray more accept the Son so they can experience Your peace and safety in a broken world. So that close to You, they may

DWELL.

In peace I will lie down and sleep, for you
alone, LORD, make me dwell in safety.

Psalm 4:8 NIV

REFUGE

Lord, I want a grateful heart so I can taste and feel
the good days.

You are never alone.

Fears will rob you of all that is good in your life.

Remember to invite God in the present moment.
Invite Him in so you can feed your faith and
starve your fears.

Dear God, deliver me from my fear of failure, my fears of the future—all the unwelcome fears in my life. Please, God, allow Your truth, purity, and goodness to deliver me. You, and only You, are my safe place, my refuge. Thank You for all You are doing and all You continue to do. Help me to hold Your hand in all I walk through. Help me, Lord, to do right by You. Hold my heart ♥ and show me only what You want me to see. Never can the wickedness in the world put me to shame, as long as I have You as my
REFUGE.

In you, LORD, I have taken refuge; let me never be
put to shame; deliver me in your righteousness.

Psalm 31:1 NIV

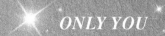

ONLY YOU

God, You are so good. According to Your Word,
YOU will remove those who deprive the innocent of justice.
YOU will . . .

Vanish the ruthless.

Make the mockers disappear.

Cut down all who have
an eye for evil.

Lord, my hope is in You. My faith is in You. My strength is in You.
And my love is in You. I know change, power, and peace will come
to those whose lives are with You. And there is much in this world
too heavy for us to carry on our own. There is much in this world too
powerful for us to fight on our own.

Dear God, I pray for broken hearts all over the world. I pray against
systemic forms of evil that oppress Your people! I pray for peace to
fill the hearts and minds of Your people, and I pray for unity in You.
Unity in Your love. In Jesus' name, I pray against the strongholds
of evil that dwell in this world and in people. They are no longer
welcomed near Your people. Your light is much stronger. I pray for
wisdom to fall from above and for justice. Lord, raise Your people
to power in all forms, all areas, so the love in their hearts will

guide them. Allowing them to rule and defend, making Your people, Your will, unstoppable. With Your love, dear Lord, all things are possible. Do what only You can do, *ONLY YOU.*

The ruthless will vanish, the mockers will disappear, and all who have an eye for evil will be cut down—those who with a word make someone out to be guilty, who ensnare the defender in court and with false testimony deprive the innocent of justice.

Isaiah 29:20-21 NIV

JUNE

PAINT YOUR LIFE

Allow Me to paint your life
I will add color, I will make it vibrant
Allow Me to paint
Allow Me to create

How do I let You, the Creator of all, paint my life?

In order for Me to paint your life,
I need full control over
the colors and the design
You must trust
My taste
My skill set
My vision

How do I let go and trust You more?

Be present with Me
You are at your happiest
when you are present because
You live in the timeline I created for your life
My timeline is divine and will never come again

Dear God, help me to trust You more with my life. Help me to trust Your vision for my life. Help me to be present, Lord, so the sufferings of today do not follow me into tomorrow. Father, keep me in perfect peace. God, I pray for more peace from above.

We are all connected, so more peace from You is more peace for me, which is more peace for people I meet and greet. The more peace You create in us, the more we trust. Then You pick up the brush and You begin to paint; as we trust You with each and every choice, every color, and every stroke, You start to create a masterpiece of Your design . . . Oh, it's divine, so please take my canvas and paint Your vision for me, a reflection of You I will be! Please, please create, Lord, in me a masterpiece, one that points to the life of the Son! Lord, You did just that. You painted His life and I hope You will do something similar with me. I forever belong to You, so use me, Lord, and make it of Your design, and in me

PAINT YOUR LIFE.

You will keep in perfect peace those whose minds
are steadfast, because they trust in you.

Isaiah 26:3 NIV

I HEAR, I SEE, I MOVE

Vendy, you think I do not know
the cries of My people?
You think I am so removed?
You think I cannot hear them or see them?
You think I cannot hear or see you?

The Lord gives bread of adversity
and water of affliction.

What is happening now, I use for good
What happened then, I use for good
I am just in a way no man can be just
I am all-seeing and all-knowing

Evil is real.

How do we overcome evil?

We become more like God.

As for you, you meant evil against me, but God meant
it for good in order to bring about this present result,
to preserve many people alive.

Genesis 50:20 NASB 1995

God, how do we be more like You?

To be like God is to hear the
cries of many.

In quietness and trust, God gives strength. God can stop the world and raise up His people. He uses all things for your good, and He will rise up to show compassion to the world.

I give strength, come to Me in trust and be still

Dear Lord, You are just in a way that no human can ever be just. You long to be gracious to me and You have always risen up to meet me with compassion, even during the times I did not choose You. Lord, because of this, because of Your forgiving hand, help me to do the same for others. Father, help me to wait on You. And then, only then, when it is from You, will
I HEAR, I SEE, I MOVE.

Yet the LORD longs to be gracious to you; therefore he
will rise up to show you compassion. For the LORD is
a God of justice. Blessed are all who wait for him!

Isaiah 30:18 NIV

NOBLE PLANS

What side of history do you want to be on? What character in the movie do you want to be?

God, help us move. Help Your people take action, help them be part of Your change so we can stand together with noble plans.

God makes us part of His army by growing our
hearts in love and compassion, growing our
hearts in empathy.

LORD, be gracious to us; we long for you. Be our strength
every morning, our salvation in time of distress.

Isaiah 33:2 NIV

Dear Lord, be my strength and teach me what I need to do
differently in my life. How do I help Your world with my life? How
do I bring Your kingdom here? Show me the deeds and
make the plans, then help me stand firm in Your
NOBLE PLANS.

But the noble make noble plans and
by noble deeds they stand.

Isaiah 32:8 NIV

JUSTICE

Lord, I am sorry for the times I have failed to speak up.
I am sorry for the times I did speak, but lacked Your wisdom.

It takes courage to stand up for what you know
is right. It takes wisdom to deliver. One
without the other is not effective.

If we want to be successful in producing an intended result for
justice, we must be courageous enough to speak, and our words must
be paired with God's wisdom!

Dear Lord, I am sorry and I humble myself to You. Help me,
God, teach me and guide me. Please bless Your people with the
COURAGE and **WISDOM** to speak at the times we need to speak.
Lace our words with indisputable truth that opens hearts and minds
to perspectives from above. God, I pray for streams in the deserts of
this world 🌍 and for more of Your
JUSTICE.

Water will gush forth in the wilderness
and streams in the desert.

Isaiah 35:6 NIV

INCREASE

Weary: Exhausted in strength, endurance, vigor,
or freshness.

God is so powerful and so divine that He never tires. Sometimes just thinking of something that exhausts me makes me tired. Just the thought . . .

As humans, we rule the land and watch over His creation, but we are weak and limited compared to God.

God gives strength to the weary and increases the power of the weak.

When I was at my weakest, I saw the power of God in my life. What is making you weary? Where do you need an increase in strength?

Dear Father, I have heard You and I know You. You the everlasting, the beginning and the end, the mighty publisher of peace! You are the One Who gave me understanding, power, and strength when I was very weak. Father, now that I know, I must tell the world. I need Your help, I need Your angels to deliver the world these keys. These keys fell from heaven when I needed them most—when I was weary and weak. These keys increase the power of the weak and lost. Keys, Father, for those who don't know You, for those who live far from You and carry their own yokes! I can't imagine how they must feel, navigating this world without You. Oh, don't let it be true. Father, many of these souls are people I love. Many of these souls are my friends, my family.

Father, I pray for them. I want them to come to You! Father, this soul could even be my love, the one You created for me and from his rib You crafted me. Oh, Father, tell all I love, and this world, of You and Your ways so we can see an immeasurable

INCREASE.

Do you not know? Have you not heard? The LORD is the everlasting God, the Creator of the ends of the earth. He will not grow tired or weary, and his understanding no one can fathom. He gives strength to the weary and increases the power of the weak.

Isaiah 40:28-29 NIV

SERVE THE LORD

God, You establish justice.
God, You bring peace.
God, You redeem.

We will falter and be discouraged, but through
faithfulness His will can be done.

Dear Lord, today I ask for forgiveness. Where I have done wrong,
please allow Your redeeming love to enter. Where injustice has
happened to Your children, please bring healing smooth as honey
and shower the innocent. Protect the innocent. May more souls run,
sprint, race to the house of the Lord! For how could there ever be
true justice unless we serve the Creator of justice? I pray more souls
enter the house of the Lord! I pray more souls learn to
SERVE THE LORD.

In faithfulness he will bring forth justice; he will
not falter or be discouraged till he establishes
justice on earth.

Isaiah 42:3-4 NIV

YOU SEE ALL

You know each person's name
You know each person's pain
You know each person's game
You know each person's past
You know each person's present

If we trust in Him, He will make things
right in our lives.

Dear God, please grant protection. You know the flames of fire
people have had to walk through, You know the innocent that have
been robbed. You see it all. May we learn to place our trust in You
and You only. Father, my sweet sister. You know her name. You
know her pain. You know her game. You know her past. You know
her present. Father, my sister is in the hands of darkness. She was
robbed as a child. Father, don't let me grow weary in praying for
her. Father, don't let the praying mothers around the world grow
weary in lifting up their requests for their children. Father, for those
who need it the most, I pray You summon them by name. I pray
they know they belong to You, the One Who created them. When
they pass through the waters, be with them! When they pass through
the river, don't let it sweep over them. When they walk through the
fire, don't let it burn them. Father, she has been mutilated, her life
has gone up in flames. Don't let us stop, don't let my family stop,
praying for her, Father, because You know her name.
You know her pain, and
YOU SEE ALL.

Do not fear, for I have redeemed you; I have summoned you by name; you are mine.
When you pass through the waters, I will be with you; and when you pass through
the rivers, they will not sweep over you. When you walk through the fire, you will
not be burned; the flames will not set you ablaze.

Isaiah 43:1-2 NIV

MARKED LIFE

Vendy, give Me your heart 🤍
Allow Me to plant many cares
I place people in your life
I give you signs and
instincts that open your eyes
Listen
Be still
Listen

To all God's children: He wants you to know
He is always here. Always.

Vendy, I will fill your life with growth
Everywhere you go will be watered,
life will grow around you,
making all things new and green
With Me by your side,
you will bring healing, truth, and light
That cannot be turned off or shut out
I have a divine plan for your life
orchestrated by the heavens
Let Me do what only I can do
I will lace your every move, your every step,
with courage and wisdom
All you have to do is trust Me
Wait for Me
I'm never late

Dear Father, I feel it in my bones: The heavens are jumping for joy, the angels are circling Your throne, because the time has come. The training is complete in me, for I have **FINALLY** learned to trust You. To surrender to You. To wait on You. For when You move, Father, it is mighty. No weapon can prosper against Your move. So, Lord, take my many cares and turn them into dreams. Do what only You can do. Seal my lips and let it be Your Spirit that moves. May abundant life begin to flow from the knees that bend to You. Let healing, truth, and light shine from my
MARKED LIFE.

A dream comes when there are many cares, and
many words mark the speech of a fool.

Ecclesiastes 5:3 NIV

I AM FOR YOU

We are made for eternity, so our old age and our gray hairs do not change the way God sees us. Our years on earth are limited, and His view of us will always be how a loving Father views His child . . . innocent and hopeful.

He sustains us
He created us
He will carry us through all things
He sustains us

He will strengthen and support us, physically and mentally, through suffering.

Because we are like children to God, we suffer like children do. When we are in deep pain, when we cannot see what's next, when we don't trust our parent who is protecting us and teaching us, our suffering seems unbearable. When children suffer, they have zero ability to comprehend other perspectives.

The pain we experience here on earth is real. The suffering is real. But God says He will sustain us, carry us, and rescue us to our old age because to God, our human years do not compare to His eternity.

Dear God, may Your favor be upon Your people for a thousand generations. For their family and their children's children. Show people, Lord, that You are with them—all those who suffer. I pray they grow to know and feel Your Spirit with them. Father, You are for us, the suffering souls of the world. Therefore, You will sustain us and rescue us. And Lord, because You were there for my suffering soul, forever

I AM FOR YOU.

Even to your old age and gray hairs I am he, I am he who will sustain you. I have made you and I will carry you; I will sustain you and I will rescue you.

Isaiah 46:4 NIV

FATHERS LIKE AL

There is sooooo much I miss about my dad. His smile, his nature, his love, his laugh, his faith, his hopeful heart.

Fathers like Al.

None of us are perfect, but God looks at the way we love. The stance of our hearts towards others. Towards people.

There is much pain in this world because of the lack of and need for fathers.

Fathers that lead. Fathers with courage and faith. Fathers filled with love.

When people have fathers, the guidance and protection over their lives is powerful. When people don't have fathers, I believe they are at a disadvantage.

The good news is everyone is welcomed by God the Father.

Dear Lord, I pray for more loving fathers like Al, the one I had for twenty-three years. We need more fathers like Al: pure of heart, who love with You at the center. Bless this world with them. I pray that my children and their children experience my father's love because it lives in me and can be passed on through them. I pray they experience it. I pray that You may see Your children who are a long way off and run to them, wrapping Your arms around them and planting a kiss on them. God, I have experienced a world with a loving father and without one—so I know the **HUGE** difference it makes. Lord, please move in like You moved in for me and be there for those who need a Father. I pray for more *FATHERS LIKE AL.*

> But while he was still a long way off, his father saw him and was filled with compassion for him; he ran to his son, threw his arms around him and kissed him.
>
> **Luke 15:20 NIV**

REJOICE, YOU EARTH

Compassion: Sympathy and concern for the sufferings
or misfortunes of others.

🗝 Because God is full of compassion,
He brings comfort.

Comfort: A state of physical ease and freedom from pain
or constraint. Ease the grief or distress of; console.

Our sufferings on earth are only for a moment. Because we are built
for eternity, the pain we endure here is nothing but an inhale.

Dear Lord, I am so thankful for Your love and the tenderness
You brought to my life. I pray for more of Your love and comfort
everywhere. I pray for more of Your presence here on earth.
Affliction has filled my life, yet so has blessing and glory, which
almost always surpass the suffering. So today I shout for joy because
I see so clearly what You do and have done. Bring comfort and
expand our hearts . . . make a way when there is no way . . . shake
the world and flip it upside down! Yup, sounds about right. Father,
pour down Your Spirit, lower the heavens,
and tell them. Tell them all. Oh,
REJOICE, YOU EARTH!

Shout for joy, you heavens; rejoice, you earth; burst into
song, you mountains! For the LORD comforts his people
and will have compassion on his afflicted ones.

Isaiah 49:13 NIV

HOPEFUL ARM

Many things will fail us. We could lose a job, lose a loved one, and lose hope in a relationship. We can lose our joys, lose our dreams, lose our joy-filled spirits. There is nothing in this world you can place salvation in except for God.

God's salvation: Preservation or deliverance from harm, ruin, or loss.

We may experience ruin or loss, but His salvation grants deliverance from this loss. His salvation will last forever. His ways will never fail you.

My salvation will last forever
My righteousness will never fail

Because of His salvation, we can see the good in everything. Let God take care of the bad, the ill will, and hurtful intentions from others. Leave it for Him to handle. We have freedom and peace to see the good in people's hearts, and He will take care of the bad. This allows us to love more fully.

He grants permission to see the good, enjoy the good, and live in the good.

Dear Lord, I hopefully await Your will. I hopefully live Your will. Help me, and all those I love, choose You and Your will. May all

Your people experience justice by Your arm and live in the good
You create. 🤍 Let us praise Your way as we wait for Your
HOPEFUL ARM.

My righteousness draws near speedily, my salvation is on the
way, and my arm will bring justice to the nations. The islands
will look to me and wait in hope for my arm.

Isaiah 51:5 NIV

NEVER LEAVE YOU

If you only knew how close I was to you
How tight I hold on to your hand
How closely I walk next to you every day . . .
Would you still fear?
Would you still worry?
I, the Creator of all things,
all that is good

God created change. Change will come just like
the seasons. Growth stems from change.

Change births vulnerability. If you do not fully trust in God, change
is hard to walk through alone. Scary even.

God's playground for us is the unknown. When we are there,
we tend to check in with Him more often.

God's greatest desire for you is to live a life free of
worry and fear because these two things block love
from flowing and filling your life. God wants us to
know how greatly we are loved.

When you fully trust in Me,
you let me write every chapter of your life
Every page will be new, which can be scary
But since I am your author,
what do you have to fear?

Dear Lord, please write every chapter of my life. I want to walk in obedience to Your will rather than be overcome by vulnerability. When I walk with You, I move forward and travel with confidence in every direction You lead. And therein lies much freedom. 🤍 Please, Lord, I pray to hold Your hand tight and *NEVER LEAVE YOU*.

See, my servant will act wisely; he will be raised
and lifted up and highly exalted.

Isaiah 52:13 NIV

HIGHLIGHT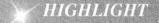

Time with You is special
It comforts my heart
It soothes my soul
It's wisdom and unexpected
It's always my highlight

Hearing from our Creator is unlike anything else.

God's thoughts ☀ are higher than our thoughts . . .
Maybe that's why His perspective is so powerful . . .

God, how do I have more of Your thoughts?

You feed yourself with My truth

How do I get more of your truth?

Just ask Me
When prayers go up, I hear every one
Your prayers are your lifeline and the
best form of communication with Me

Hearing from You is special
It comforts my heart
It soothes my soul
It's wisdom and unexpected
It's always my highlight

Dear Lord, we learn more of Your truth in Scripture, which is full of wisdom. But nothing can replace the quality time we spend with You. Our prayers, our time, our thoughts, our love—You care for these most. Father, I pray more souls surrender their thoughts and time to You. If it's close to anything I have experienced, they will quickly come to learn that quality time with You will always be their
HIGHLIGHT.

"For my thoughts are not your thoughts, neither are your ways my ways," declares the LORD. "As the heavens are higher than the earth, so are my ways higher than your ways and my thoughts than your thoughts."

Isaiah 55:8-9 NIV

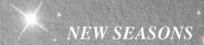

NEW SEASONS

God leads us to joy and peace. Some days are cloudy,
some nights are restless, but the results from above are
always joy, peace, and victory.

Picturing mountains, hills, or trees bursting into song or clapping
their hands is a powerful vision. Challenging to imagine, but so
clearly demonstrating the wonders of God's ways. He created the
mountains. He created the hills. He carefully placed them where they
are, and if He ascribes human qualities to His creation, who am I to
limit what God says?

If He can make mountains sing, mountains that are far
less valuable to Him than you, I can only imagine what
He can do in your life . . .

His creation will clap and sing at the glory He
will pour down into your life.

When we embody His teachings, His words flow down
from above and water us. They grow us to accomplish all
He places on our hearts—with joy and peace as a reward.

There is great purpose for what God is doing in
your life. So trust Him today. With this
moment. With what is next.

Nothing God starts in you will return empty.

Dear Lord, from Your mouth to my ears, I pray for this new season
I am entering. I pray Your promises do not return empty, for I know
the good works You started in me will be accomplished. Not for
my name's sake, but for Your glory and the glory of Your children.
Those who choose You in their

NEW SEASONS.

So is my word that goes out from my mouth: It will not return to me empty,
but will accomplish what I desire and achieve the purpose for which I sent it.
You will go out in joy and be led forth in peace; the mountains and hills will
burst into song before you, and all the trees of the field will
clap their hands.

Isaiah 55:11-12 NIV

JULY

ALL WHO NEED

How does someone's light rise in the darkness? How is God able to turn our night into noonday?

When you step outside of yourself, God uses the pain of whatever was formed against you and turns it into your greatest strength. That is how your light rises—even in complete darkness.

Loose chains of injustice
Set the oppressed free
Share your food with the hungry
Provide the poor with shelter

Where is there injustice in your life? How do you work to overcome this?

Who is hungry in your life? How do you provide food and shelter for their minds and bodies?

Dear God, I thank You for another beautiful day. I ask that You bless the hearts and minds of those who suffer and walk the night without You. Please, Lord, move in Your people's hearts to break chains of injustice and provide for
ALL WHO NEED.

And if you spend yourselves in behalf of the hungry and satisfy
the needs of the oppressed, then your light will rise in the darkness,
and your night will become like the noonday.

Isaiah 58:10 NIV

MY GARDEN

The thing about gardens is you can always tell from looking at them whether they are well kept or not. How well watered they are.

What our Creator supplies is eternal and
never-ending. He is the best gardener.
He has the ability to:

Always guide
Satisfy needs
Strengthen you
And He never fails

Dear God, please water my garden so even in sun-scorched land I can have Your peace. 🤍 Please supply your never-ending joy, peace, and love so I can always grow. Father, please continue to strengthen my frame and tend to
MY GARDEN.

The LORD will guide you always; he will satisfy your needs in a sun-scorched land and will strengthen your frame. You will be like a well-watered garden, like a spring whose waters never fail.

Isaiah 58:11 NIV

LORD HAS SPOKEN

Why do You want to be first in my life, Lord?

So I can best protect you
Vendy, when I come first,
everything that follows is a blessing,
but not your foundation

Only God is built to be your one
and only foundation.

How do I put You first? How do I make **YOU** my
foundation and not the blessings in my life?

Believe how greatly I want to bless you
When you truly believe this,
you only live in fear of Me
and nothing else

Dear Lord, thank You for protecting me. I am thankful for You. You give me irrevocable joy and make me happy. Because my joy rests now in You, You will lift me to new heights and carry me to triumph. From Your mouth, I will take the victory in every battle I face, for this to me the
LORD HAS SPOKEN.

"Then you will find your joy in the LORD, and I will cause you to ride in
triumph on the heights of the land and to feast on the inheritance
of your father Jacob." The mouth of the LORD has spoken.

Isaiah 58:14 NIV

EXPRESSION OF LOVE

Tenderhearted: Having a kind, gentle, or sentimental nature.

God loves me first. God loves me perfectly. We are an expression of the love we receive. When we love others well, we are an expression of God.

There is not a time in my life where I regret showing another human love. Showing a friend love. Showing someone who hurt me love. If anything, it has granted me freedom.

What does love look like?

Choosing kindness always and placing it before hurt.

God has never stopped loving me 🤍, even though I have made decisions that have hurt Him. My family loves me and my friends love me. I have been hurt by both, but I don't stop loving them.

My God, what is the key to loving like You?

Forgive

How much?

> "Lord, how often shall my brother sin against me, and I forgive him? As many as seven times?" Jesus said to him, "I do not say to you seven times, but seventy times seven."

Matthew 18:21-22 RSV

Dear Lord, why is forgiveness **SO** hard for me? I know
You instruct us to forgive seventy times seven, which is 490 times,
but that feels like such a high number. I find it easier to forgive
the people I love, so the key to forgiving others must be love. But
how do I love those who are not my family and friends? Kindness
maybe? Showing them kindness even when it is hard for me? Yes,
that's it, Lord. I will move and act in kindness because You are
always kind to me, and I am forgiven by You. So who am I to not
forgive? I pray for more forgiveness and kindness to fill this earth
so we may be like Christ, an

EXPRESSION OF LOVE.

Be kind to one another, tenderhearted, forgiving one
another, as God in Christ forgave you.

Ephesians 4:32 ESV

LIPS OF YOUR CHILDREN

Do I believe in God's goodness? Do I believe in God's rich, never-ending love? Do I believe He wants to bless His children, the way any loving parent would?

All sin is birthed out of disbelief.

When we don't believe in the promises and ways of God, we choose a path that is based on our perspective and not knowledge from above.

God has blessings for you. When you choose Him, He brings blessings to you and generations on generations.

Yes, blessings on the lips of your children and on the lips of their children.

Dear God, please help me believe in the powers that flow from above so I can stay rooted on Your path. Fill me with belief in You, Your ways, and Your truth so I can live a life full of wonders. Lord, rid me of my disbelief and bless the lips of my children. I know this belief will bring honor to generations to come. For the blessings on the lips of my children are blessings on the *LIPS OF YOUR CHILDREN.*

"As for me, this is my covenant with them," says the LORD. "My Spirit, who is on you, will not depart from you, and my words that I have put in your mouth will always be on your lips, on the lips of your children and on the lips of their descendants—from this time on and forever," says the LORD.

Isaiah 59:21 NIV

SURROUNDED BY YOU

The Lord loves justice
The Lord hates robbery and wrongdoing
For God to hate something must make it pretty bad

To counter the spirit of heaviness, put on the
garment of praise.

God says, in His faithfulness, He will reward
His people. Not in the faithfulness of the world, not in
your faithfulness or my faithfulness, but in
His faithfulness.

Vendy, let Me surround you
Invite Me into every area
And praise Me because
the battle is now in My hands

Dear Lord, I thank You for Your faithfulness. For now I can rest
because the battle is in Your hands. I gave it a few rounds and am
proud to fight for justice, but, Father, I am ready to step out of the
ring and praise my way to victory. I am ready to see You reward
Your people, the ones who have stepped out of the ring and invited
You into every area. The ones who let You surround them.
The ones who are
SURROUNDED BY YOU.

For I, the LORD, love justice; I hate robbery and wrongdoing.
In my faithfulness I will reward my people and make an
everlasting covenant with them.

Isaiah 61:8 NIV

TO BE PRAISED

The kindness of God
The deeds of God
Are never-ending

Enjoy every moment I have blessed you with
Not because every moment is peaceful,
but because it will never come again
You can choose to see your life with Me,
the great author writing every chapter,
or you can
Choose to see your life without Me
That part, I have no control over, sweet V

God does not need us to praise Him for His good deeds.
God does not need us for anything. We need God to live
our fullest, most abundant lives. A life filled with kindness
and the good deeds of God is a life lived in the present.
It's a life filled with trust and faith, even on your darkest
nights. Because with God, you have a bright light shining
in the darkness. And with God, your cup overflows.

He does not need us to choose Him, but it brings God
great joy when we do. When He sees His creation live
their fullest lives, the God of the heavens is pleased.

Dear Lord, help us see our lives with You as our author, so that with
every high and low we can continue to trust in the higher power that

is weaving it all together for our good. So we can trust You and not all we see. So Your Spirit will continue to be our guide and keep us on Your path. Oh, Father, You are worthy, so worthy, always *TO BE PRAISED.*

> I will tell of the kindnesses of the Lord, the deeds for which
> he is to be praised, according to all the Lord has done for
> us—yes, the many good things.

Isaiah 63:7 NIV

PERSONAL GUIDE

I want the entire picture. I want the roadmap to my life with exact directions for every turn. I want to know the timing and how long it will take to get to my next destination. Yes, I would like to know both the departing and arriving times along with the destination address and the number of miles to the destination. Please.

Unfortunately, this is not how God operates. He does not paint a picture for your life and show you. Rather, if you allow, His Holy Spirit accompanies you at every turn. He directs your every step. And since His hand made all things, there are no surprises for God—just for us!

God's Spirit as a personal GPS is much better than a map for your life.

As fears, worries, and doubts arise, give them to God.

He will take them lovingly and keep you on the right track.

Dear Lord, You show me glimpses of the plans You have for me, then You ask that I trust in You to see them through. You speak to the desires of my heart and act as my guide. For this, I will be forever grateful. Forever grateful for the ways You deal with me. Because I choose You, seek You, and spend time with You, I hear more clearly from You. You are able to show and tell me things

I would normally not see or understand. So today, Lord,
I continue to pray for Your divine power and will to be done on
earth. Father, I thank You for being my
PERSONAL GUIDE.

"Has not my hand made all these things, and
so they came into being?" declares the LORD.

Isaiah 66:2 NIV

TODAY I APPOINT

God, touch my mouth and put Your words in me. Fill me with
Your truth.

Today God appoints all His children to walk in His truth. The same
truth that was planted and has encouraged people
for generations.

God's truth tears down nations of all kinds of evil.

God's truth builds and grows all that is good, birthing
peace and joy.

Dear Lord, use me to build and to plant   , to overthrow evil and
nurture only good. Only what is from You. Make me into a master
gardener, a master planter! Place Your words in my mouth and direct
me when to speak and when to hold my words. Show me how to
build and how to shepherd these buildings. God, free Your believers,
Your people, and fill this earth with them so they may rule nations
and kingdoms. There is new authority I am now walking in, so
TODAY I APPOINT.

Then the Lord reached out his hand and touched my mouth and said
to me, "I have put my words in your mouth. See, today I appoint you
over nations and kingdoms to uproot and tear down, to destroy
and overthrow, to build and to plant."

Jeremiah 1:9-10 NIV

HEALING

Healing, My sweet daughter
Healing through My love
Through My light
Through My warmth
Through My touch
Through My words
Through My people
Through our time
Through your prayer
Healing, My sweet daughter

I will write every chapter
I will teach you all you need to know
I will heal you and
place you on mountaintops,
for I will never forsake you
I will always be your spring of living water
Abundance will follow you everywhere

Healing from above is the best kind. It not only
brings life back to you, but to others as well.

Vendy, let Me first bring healing
so I can bless you
in every way, shape, and form

Dear Lord, I pray healing over all who need it. I thank You for the healing from above, and I pray that You direct faithful steps for my life. I pray for faithfulness to You for all Your sweet love. Thank You for pouring out over my life streams of living water filled with *HEALING.*

Heal me, LORD, and I will be healed; save me
and I will be saved, for you are the one I praise.

Jeremiah 17:14 NIV

SHEPHERDS FROM ABOVE

How do we lead one another in the right direction?
Towards love and freedom? Towards all that is
good and from above?

A man is knowledgeable, but lacks wisdom. A woman is wise, but
lacks knowledge.

What is knowledge without understanding? What is knowledge
without wisdom to follow?

God creates shepherds in people who are after
His heart. 🤍 The best leaders have both God's
knowledge and understanding, resulting in
wisdom that builds up.

Dear Lord, I pray for more shepherds that lead, more shepherds
that are after Your heart because people are filled after walking with
them. I pray for shepherds that are courageous and strong in You.
I pray for shepherds to bless Your women. I pray for shepherds to
bless Your men. I pray for shepherds that strengthen each other.
Father, I pray for more
SHEPHERDS FROM ABOVE. 🙏

Then I will give you shepherds after my own heart, who
will lead you with knowledge and understanding.

Jeremiah 3:15 NIV

GRATEFUL

God~May You always come first. May Your voice
always be the loudest. May Your glory
fill this earth.

Relationships~The blessings are never-ending,
filled with love, kindness, experience,
wisdom, and bliss.

Appear~In all places and fill us all.

Truth~Without it, this life would lack all
color and flavor.

Eternity~Our time here is so temporary. May we
see the fullness in all life's events. They strengthen
our souls for what was created and never ends.

Fruitful~May the fruits of God's Spirit bless you
and all that you love.

Unique~God has a unique plan for your life.
May we embrace His plan and not compare
our story to others, for there is much
greatness in store for each of us.

Life~Filled with beauty each morning. Breeze
from the wind, green growing all around, and
blue in the sky.

Today I am G~R~A~T~E~F~U~L.

Dear Lord, thankful, grateful You make me! The peace of the Son rules in my heart and is new with each rising sun. Richly Your Spirit dwells in me. I am not a teacher, but hungry for You, I am. On fire for You, I am. Amazed by You, I am. My mind and heart are thankful. May You always rule me. Use me, take me where You want me to go, and let me love who You want me to love. I will serve and do all You want me to do because You have transformed my heart. I am

GRATEFUL.

And let the peace of Christ rule in your hearts, to which indeed you were called in one body. And be thankful. Let the word of Christ dwell in you richly, teaching and admonishing one another in all wisdom, singing psalms and hymns and spiritual songs, with thankfulness in your hearts to God. And whatever you do, in word or deed, do everything in the name of the Lord Jesus, giving thanks to God the Father through him.

Colossians 3:15-17 ESV

TO KNOW ME

What power is there in knowing God?

When you know what the Creator of the
universe delights in, you know what to
fill your life with.

What does the Lord delight in?

Kindness
Justice
Righteousness

The Creator of all things finds **JOY** in
something as simple as kindness.

The Creator of all things exercises justice.

The Creator of all things is righteous.

Dear Lord, today I would like to be more kind. More kind to myself
and others. I pray for justice in Your world and righteous thoughts
and actions to flow from my mind, lips, and steps. I know, because
of Your view from above, I can trust in Your wisdom and love. I pray
for more understanding to know You—Your true nature and Your
fullness—because there lies kindness, justice, and righteousness for
all people. 🤍 Oh, Father, I pray for a world where more souls walk,
move, and speak with hearts and minds that desire to know You.

Father, I also know I will get to the gates—we all will one day—and You might say to me, *Sweet V, job well done. You lived a life that reflected my Son. To live a life like Him is* TO KNOW ME.

This is what the LORD says: "Let not the wise boast of their wisdom or the strong boast of their strength or the rich boast of their riches, but let the one who boasts boast about this: that they have the understanding to know me, that I am the LORD, who exercises kindness, justice and righteousness on earth, for in these I delight," declares the LORD.

Jeremiah 9:23-24 NIV

HOPE IN OUR CREATOR

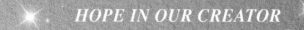

You created the sun to rise and the rain to fall
You created the birds to sing and the wind to blow
You created me
It's Your breath in my lungs

Why do I ever look to find happiness outside of You?
Why is my thinking so simple, my faith so little?

Is it not Your creation that points to the heavens?
Are we not of Your design? So then, let us place
our hope in You, the master designer of all.

Dear God, I pray for more faith. I see Your wonders in creation
every day. I wake up to their sounds and beautiful sights. Yet my
faith is so small. My faith is weak compared to Your many wonders.
The many ways You work in my life and in the lives of those around
me. Help me to place all—not some, but **ALL**—of my hope in You.
Your ways. Your will. 🤍 Please, God, help us place all our
HOPE IN OUR CREATOR.

Do the skies themselves send down showers? No, it is you,
Lord our God. Therefore our hope is in you, for you are
the one who does all this.

Jeremiah 14:22 NIV

WAVES MOVE

Do you see the way the waves move?
Do you see the water crash on the rocks?
Do you see then the sun slide down the sky and
the water calm?

This is the movement of your life
Just as the waters move,
so do joys and pains, highs and lows
I am here to tell you that I am truly above it all
So invite Me in, and ride each wave
Know that the sun always sets and rises
Know that I am at the center of it and your praise
and trust in Me determines your joy each day
Not the state of the sea ~ not the current

What do you trust God with the most?
What do you trust God with the least?
And where will you invite Him in?

Dear Lord, the tides change, and with them so do the waves.
I am learning to ride each wave with You. Some days I am much
better at this than others, but I am learning to bring my anxieties to
You. After my prayer and praise, I can then move with an

understanding that transcends due to the view You give. Father, guard the hearts and minds of the innocent and teach them how to navigate a world that feels so far from You at times. Teach them, teach us, Lord, the many ways the
WAVES MOVE.

Do not be anxious about anything, but in every situation, by prayer and petition, with thanksgiving, present your requests to God. And the peace of God, which transcends all understanding, will guard your hearts and your minds in Christ Jesus.

Philippians 4:6-7 NIV

MY POWER AND MIGHT

How does God teach us His power and His might?

We, as humans, like to create gods. We put our hope, identity, and praise in things that fade . . . our careers, relationships, and so on. Then you lose a job, a family member passes—where you once found comfort and love is suddenly gone.

God showed me His power and might when I lost my dad.

I know there is an all-powerful Lord because He taught me His power and might when my world 🌍 fell apart.

Sometimes it's good for things in our lives to fall apart. It gives God an opportunity to teach us of His power and might.

Dear Lord, I know Your strength because I have seen it work in my life. I have created many false gods over the past twenty-five years, so I pray to keep You first. 🤍 I pray for all of us here on earth to see Your glory by removing our false gods. Your ways are higher than our ways and Your thoughts ☁️ are higher than our thoughts. Please fill Your people's minds and teach them of Your power and might. I know Your name: Your name is Lord. You have sent King Jesus, and because of Him, I am new. From You and through Him is *MY POWER AND MIGHT.*

"Do people make their own gods? Yes, but they are not gods!"
"Therefore I will teach them—this time I will teach them my power and might. Then they will know that my name is the LORD."

Jeremiah 16:20-21 NIV

BLESSED WHO TRUST

Why are we called to trust in God?

He calls us to do scary things—things that go against our ways of thinking. Things that go against our feelings.

If my confidence is in God . . . then I am always confident because He never fails me.

It's hard to have confidence in something you don't trust.

When we trust God, we are blessed. When our confidence is in Him, our worries fade, we overcome our fears, and—despite the climate—we are fruitful.

Dear Lord, please help me to keep You first. Please help me to trust in You. Please help me to place my confidence in You. Please, Lord, I only want to bear Your fruits. Guide my each step. And please, God, grant peace along the way. May our leaves always be green with You, *BLESSED WHO TRUST.*

But blessed is the one who trusts in the LORD, whose confidence is in him. They will be like a tree planted by the water that sends out its roots by the stream. It does not fear when heat comes; its leaves are always green. It has no worries in a year of drought and never fails to bear fruit.

Jeremiah 17:7-8 NIV

LIVING WATER

Sanctuary: A place of refuge or safety.

My sanctuary is created when I have time alone with God. It could be in the mornings with my coffee or at the beach looking out at the ocean. No matter where it is, I have a slice of bliss and peace.

Where is your sanctuary?

A glorious throne, exalted from the beginning,
is the place of our sanctuary.

Jeremiah 17:12 NIV

God wants us to come to Him. He wants to give us
hints about where He is taking us to keep us going
and to encourage us! He enjoys sharing hopes for
what He has planned with His creation.

Dear God, I am grateful for the space You hold in my life. I pray for more of it. I pray more of Your people create a glorious throne for You in their lives, so they can experience abundant peace amid suffering. Or abundant peace in the unknown. Or abundant love in the middle of confusion. Lord, may more living water spring from Your people's sanctuaries everywhere. 🤍 My God, You have healed me and saved me, so forever I will praise You. Grateful, I am, for the streams that flow from my pain, the
LIVING WATER.

Heal me, LORD, and I will be healed; save me and
I will be saved, for you are the one I praise.

Jeremiah 17:14 NIV

THINK PRAISEWORTHY

Do miracles have to happen in your life to praise God?

Do good or great things have to happen for you to praise God?

Truthfully, even on my worst days, there are many praiseworthy
blessings to give thanks for. But I rarely do. Why?

It's easy to look to God when things do not go as planned, but I
know He'd like to teach me more on the power of praise.

Sweet V, there is power in praise

When we keep grateful hearts and praise Him
through the highs and lows, we live lives filled
with peace. Our praise is not because God needs
it, it's for our minds. It's for our transformation.
It's for our lives. It's for our belief!

Where do I start, God?

Thank Me for all I've done,
and for what I will continue to do
Thank Me for how I'm going to
work good out of everything that hurts you
Out of all of the things you cannot control
Smile, laugh, and thank Me again
Thank Me for our time
Thank Me for the love in your life
Thank Me for the protection
over your life

Dear Lord, there is not one thing in my life from You that is not praiseworthy. You plant truths. Help me crave what is noble, right, pure, and lovely. You help me honor what is admirable, and You bless me with perfect peace. I wonder what this world would look like if we all thought about things that are excellent and praiseworthy? Lord, I wonder how the atmosphere would shift? I wonder what it would look like for You to flip the script! Father, may Your presence go before people—believers and nonbelievers—and show them how to

THINK PRAISEWORTHY.

Finally, brothers and sisters, whatever is true, whatever is noble, whatever is right, whatever is pure, whatever is lovely, whatever is admirable—if anything is excellent or praiseworthy—think about such things.

Philippians 4:8 NIV

STRENGTH OF MY HEART

Vendy, things will not always appear as you imagine
But that's because I can do far more than you imagine

When God is at the center of my heart 🤍, all love flows evenly
and smoothly. Similar to the way veins supply fresh blood from
our hearts to our organs, when God is at the center, we operate in
balance. The way He designed us.

My vital organs are the people I love most—my family and friends.
The veins carry equal amounts to the people who need it most in my
life. It is fluid and balanced.

Our Creator is so divine. Much thought went into
creating us. Our bodies and souls are divine, and
when nourished, they operate at full capacity.

I want to love at full capacity, and I know, for me, the only way
I can truly do this is if God is at the center.

Dear Lord, please help me keep You first so I can operate at full
capacity for myself and others. ⚔️ My fleshy heart may fail, but
You are the
STRENGTH OF MY HEART.

My flesh and my heart may fail, but God is the strength
of my heart and my portion forever.

Psalm 73:26 NIV

ALL WENT WELL ✦

What does it mean to know God?

By faith, we move in directions that make sense
in God's eyes and not in the eyes of this world.

By faith, we do things we don't always want to
do . . . out of compassion and love for God.

When we care enough to move, God sees . . . and all will go
well for you. 🩶

Dear Lord, there are many causes placed on my heart,
but I do not always make them a priority. Help me love
the needy and broken in my life better. Similar to how
You loved me in my brokenness. Please, Lord, always tend to my
neediness. I pray, God, that Your people grow to know You so
intimately that it causes them to defend the people who need it
the most. Oh, Father, only with You can I say,
"ALL WENT WELL."

"He defended the cause of the poor and needy, and so
all went well. Is that not what it means to know me?"
declares the LORD.

Jeremiah 22:16 NIV

FILL HEAVEN AND EARTH

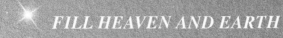

Is it possible to hide from God?
I don't think so.

Then why do we try so hard to hide our desires from Him?

I wish My people knew how greatly I desire to bless them

Many times the desires that live in our hearts
are from God. The blessings He'd like to pour
over you sometimes take longer because we are
not ready. We are not prepared for the greatness
God has in store, for the many mighty
plans—because we make the blessings our
gods. When we worship the blessings from
Him, He no longer comes first.

Time and time again this happens to me. I need God's help in
keeping Him first in my heart. That way I have joy in all things, and
my blessings don't become false gods I begin to worship.

Dear Lord, You fill the heavens and the earth with all that is good.
All blessings stem from above. They come from You. My sweet
God, thank You for Your goodness and all You have done. Please
help me be more in love with You over anything You bless me with.
After all, who else can

FILL HEAVEN AND EARTH?

"Am I only a God nearby," declares the LORD, "and not a God far away?
Who can hide in secret places so that I cannot see them?" declares
the LORD. "Do not I fill heaven and earth?" declares the LORD.

Jeremiah 23:23-24 NIV

AUGUST

CONTINUED LOVE

Great love
New every morning
Compassion and faithfulness

The Lord is good to those whose hope is in Him.

What does that look like?

Patience. Continued gratitude through the good and the bad, the old and the new. Persistent and continued love showcased through obedience to His ways, which are higher than our own.

His love is the greatest we can experience on earth. It's new every morning and filled with compassion and faithfulness that pours and spills over into all areas of our lives. It makes us new, strong, joy-filled, and peaceful.

Dear Lord, help us to wait hopefully for Your will! The portions that flow from above move mountains, bless us, and keep our minds sound. May I always seek You and wait quietly for You. Thank You, Lord, for Your
CONTINUED LOVE.

Because of the LORD's great love we are not consumed, for his compassions never fail. They are new every morning; great is your faithfulness. I say to myself, "The LORD is my portion; therefore I will wait for him." The LORD is good to those whose hope is in him, to the one who seeks him; it is good to wait quietly for the salvation of the LORD.

Lamentations 3:22-26 NIV

MY WORDS

Vendy, I want My people to know
that I'm always here
I may seem far
Your mind may get clouded with thoughts
that make it harder to hear from Me
But I'm always here
Close your door, find a quiet space,
Talk to Me
Lay with Me
Process with Me
Let Me bless you with
wisdom for the problems you wrestle with
Let Me guide you
Let Me do it all
You were not made
to navigate this world on your own
You live your best life with Me by your side,
living close to Me and praising Me

Please, invite Him in.

God can do wonders if we just invite Him in. If we can just spend time with Him. Give more to Him. Be vulnerable with Him. Trust Him. Believe in Him. He can do so much.

Dear Lord, help me invite You into every area of my life. 🤍 May Your words be the first I tend to. Allow them to guide my steps. Do what You must to tenderize my heart. May Your words become the foundation for my life. God, my flesh is weak, but Your promises keep me going, they fill me. I hope to reflect You. I pray to live a life that reflects You. May Your words become
MY WORDS.

It is the Spirit who gives life; the flesh is no help at all.
The words that I have spoken to you are
spirit and life.

John 6:63 ESV

WHO I AM

Vendy, I want you to have joy,
joy abundantly, because of Who I am
Not because things go according to how you'd like
But because of Who I am
I am the One that will strengthen
and support you—physically and mentally

Friends, family, readers . . . He will sustain you.
Just turn to Him. Look up! He will always
be there for you.

Dear Lord, some days I feel Your strength carrying me through—
especially the tough days. Thank You for the support and strength
You have provided. 🤍 Help me to see this, to know this, and believe
this on all days. May joy come purely from knowing and believing
in Your goodness. Thank You for another day; I pray You continue to
write each one. With You, I love
WHO I AM.

I am he who will sustain you.

Isaiah 46:4 NIV

LET PAIN IN

The older we get, the more we see and experience on our journey through life. I could be hurt by someone, or I could hurt someone. Rather than face the pain, thinking I am helping myself, I will choose to pretend the pain isn't there. Suffering and pain come in many different forms; pain is universal and all humans will experience it in some form while on earth.

Pain turned over to God grows our hearts.

Why do you want God to grow your heart?

So you can live a life full of love.

Why is love important or special?

Because a life without love is empty and colorless.

Dear Lord, I notice I'm a much better person when I experience pain with You. I have compassion. I can be present and there for people I love. I don't like this, but pain has taught me a lot. It's taught me how much I need You and how empty a life without love is. I pray to take the pain in every area of my life and hand it over to You so I can love more fully and be there for people I care for the way You have been there for me. Father, with You, we can
LET PAIN IN.

He heals the brokenhearted and binds up their wounds.

Psalm 147:3 NIV

DELIGHT IN MERCY

Mercy: Compassion or forgiveness shown toward
someone who is within one's power to punish or harm.

At one point or another, we have all been in a situation where we
had a choice to show compassion and mercy or stay upset
and angry.

The times I chose to stay angry ended up
robbing me of my peace.

When we are hopeful through life events and towards people,
leading from a place of love, we are more inclined to show mercy.

How powerful is mercy towards others if the heart's desire of the
Creator of all things is to show mercy?

Dear God, bless me with a heart 🤍 that delights to show mercy, like
You! Lord, mercy is of and from You. It points to the heavens, and
we all need it because we all fall so short. A world without it would
be a scary, dark place. Father, may we learn to forgive because it was
You Who forgave first. May we
DELIGHT IN MERCY.

You do not stay angry forever but delight to show mercy.

Micah 7:18 NIV

BRING YOU BACK

Call on Me
Pray to Me
Seek Me
Find Me

The Lord will free you from captivity.

Captivity: The condition of being imprisoned or confined.

Captivity of your mind
Captivity of your actions
Captivity of your heart
Captivity of your life

Free: The state of not being imprisoned or enslaved.

When we run to God, He is there. When we
pray to God, He listens. When we seek Him
with all our heart, He shows up.

I find myself in this pattern with God often. He leads me to
acceptance in mysterious ways. Acceptance that life will not always
go as planned. Just when I think I know what is around the corner,
God moves. His ways are mysterious—difficult or impossible to
understand, explain, or identify!

His understanding is inscrutable.

Dear Lord, help me to trust in You with all my heart and mind. You dwell much higher than I do. I do not have the answers, but You do. I pray to move with You and not my flesh. Please, God, help me lean on You and trust the direction You pave for me. Father, I pray You never grow tired of bringing me back. I may choose chains . . . Whenever I do not choose You, Lord, I choose captivity! Please never grow tired of bringing me back, for I will always want to belong to You. Please, will You promise me this?

Please, please, just say, *Sweet V, I will always BRING YOU BACK.*

"Then you will call on me and come and pray to me, and I will listen to you. You will seek me and find me when you seek me with all your heart. I will be found by you," declares the LORD, "and will bring you back from captivity."

Jeremiah 29:12-14 NIV

WRITE TO ME

I do not consider myself a writer, but I write nearly every day. It's been one of the most healing things in my life, and I believe the encouragement to write came from above.

Writing to God heals.

Writing out my prayers gives me clarity. It helps me grow deeper in my faith because I can document God's words and then look back at how He has moved. How things I have prayed about have come to form. Or how things I haven't prayed about, but He has told me, came to fruition.

Our minds race and get clogged with thoughts that don't always help us.

Writing out what is heavy on
your mind and heart will
help you discern truth from lies.

We live in a world where constant reminders of truth will allow you to live a full life. Reminders of your identity.
Your worth. Your love.

Dear Lord, I write to You now throughout all seasons of my life because I love to see the powerful ways You move. I love to date my letters and journal entries to You. That way, when doubt or disbelief washes over me or those I care for, all I have to do is pick up a book! Oh, the power You ascribe to the simple things! Father, You have restored me, so I will forever write to You because I love all You place on my heart. I love the words You *WRITE TO ME*.

Write in a book all the words that I have spoken to you.
For behold, days are coming, declares the LORD, when
I will restore . . .

Jeremiah 30:2-3 ESV

BLESSINGS OF TODAY

Help me, Lord, open my eyes to the blessings of today
Help me see the green outside my window
Help me taste my warm cup of matcha
Help me pray for others and not just myself
Help me, Lord, experience the blessings of today, for
I know today will never come again

God will help you enjoy the blessings of today.

Help me lead with love today
Help me be present today
Help me care for another human today
Help me see You all around me today

Dear Lord, Your goodness is new every day and I do not always choose to see it. I remember praying for what I have today, so please, Lord, help me enjoy it. With You, there is still so much more to come. Shine Your face upon me and give me peace. Bless and keep me, Lord. Father, I pray more eyes be opened to the *BLESSINGS OF TODAY.*

The LORD bless you and keep you; The LORD make his
face to shine upon you, And be gracious to you; The LORD
lift up his countenance upon you and give you peace.

Numbers 6:24-26 NKJV

BEST RELATIONSHIP

Just spending a little time with Me
changes the shape of your heart

It's such an unbalanced relationship. God, I'm always coming to You
with all my stuff. How are You?
What can I do for You?

Love Me

How?

Choose Me . . .

But that's good for me . . . ?
Not for your benefit.

I know 😊

A relationship with our Creator is the best relationship to be in. He
has a never-ending supply of love and wealth of all sorts that feeds
you. And although it's a very uneven relationship to be in (God
does all the giving), it makes Him smile, and there's nothing He'd
like more than to be in relationship with us. He wants to be the first
person we process with. He wants to be the person we empty
our hearts 🩶 and minds to.

I will never understand why God desires to be in a relationship with me. I bring far less to the table, but that's the nature of His goodness. He just wants to see us full and complete. And the only way we can live as full and complete beings is with Him.

The best relationship you can pour into is the one from above. This relationship will feed and grow you so you can discover harmony with others.

Sometimes I don't always run to God first because He doesn't feel as close as my family or friends. All I have to do is pick up the phone or get in my car with them, but the truth is He is always there and more eager to bear fruit in our lives than we could possibly understand.

Diligent: In a way that shows care and conscientiousness in one's work or duties.

Dear Lord, help us to seek you diligently because it's the *BEST RELATIONSHIP.*

I am the vine, you are the branches; the one who remains in Me, and I in him bears much fruit, for apart from Me you can do nothing.

John 15:5 NASB

RETURN TO ME

Let Me love you with all My heart so you will overflow
Let today be from Me
Believe today is from Me

Vendy . . .

Lay down your career at My feet
Lay down your friendships at My feet
Lay down your family at My feet
Lay down your desires at My feet

Now trust Me
Do you trust Me?

We were not built to journey alone. There's
too much to be done. Too many in need. It
doesn't matter who you are, we will all fall
short again and again without God.

The good news? We have an all-powerful, redeeming God 🤍
Who sprinkles grace everywhere.

Redeeming: Compensating for someone's or something's
faults; compensatory.

Dear Lord, thank You for Your redeeming love over me. Help me to move through life with this love towards others. You have swept away my sins like a morning mist. I will continue to return to You because Your love is the most freeing and redeeming thing there is. Father, it is You I love. Please accept me and all I thought I lost by bending a knee to You, or all I thought I lost in the pain—my carefree nature, friends, and dreams—please

RETURN TO ME.

> I have swept away your offenses like a cloud, your sins like
> the morning mist. Return to me, for I have redeemed you.

Isaiah 44:22 NIV

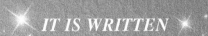 *IT IS WRITTEN*

When I think of Jesus . . .

Humility . . . Full of life . . . Suffering . . .
Comforter . . . Giving

These are the words that come to mind when I think of Jesus, God's
Son. Jesus is also God, but Jesus was also fully human. I don't
understand this completely and I might never, but I do believe it.

Jesus dealt with everything we did. He fought the desires of His
flesh. Even though He was God, He lived as fully human. As a
human, He was tempted in the same ways we are tempted.

What did Jesus do to stay strong?

Jesus went to the Father and prayed.

Jesus knew God's words, which are found in Scripture.

Those are two very powerful actions. Prayer
is communication—your lifeline to the
heavens. Knowing God's words will help you
choose life and truth instead of death
and harmful things.

Sometimes truth means choosing something that
doesn't bring you comfort in the moment, but you
know is right. We are weak; at times, to our flesh,
it feels right to choose comfort over truth. Knowing
God's words will guide and protect your steps.

Dear Lord, I shall not live by bread alone, but by Your living words that are written in Your Holy Book. In the Holy Book lives the words from the mouth of God. From the mouth of God is truth that cuts down lies and sets captives free! Freedom in mind, heart, and soul. Freedom freedom freedom flows from the lips of the Creator Who says,

"IT IS WRITTEN"!

Then Jesus was led up by the Spirit into the wilderness to be tempted by the devil. And when He had fasted forty days and forty nights, afterward He was hungry. Now when the tempter came to Him, he said, "If You are the Son of God, command that these stones become bread." But He answered and said, "It is written, 'Man shall not live by bread alone, but by every word that proceeds from the mouth of God.'"

Matthew 4:1-4 NKJV

YOUR TIME

There is a time for everything in life. By God's good will, may you experience all things in His divine time.

The Lord has a delightful timeline for all of us. He is the beginning and the end. He knows our thoughts before we do. He knows our actions before they happen.

It is possible to experience things that are not in His divine timeline due to free will. We choose. We all have choices.

When our life experiences follow God's timeline, we flourish. We find healing in His time. We reap a harvest in His time.

What happens when our life experiences occur outside of God's timeline?

Oftentimes we are not ripe. (**Ripe:** Developed to the point of readiness for harvesting.) The blessing He so greatly wanted to bestow will not keep. We are not fully matured. The healing has not finished. The work has not been completed. The confusion stays. The lies make a home and the truth is contorted.

God's timeline for your life is so rich and full of all that is good. When your life happens in His will, the glory of the Lord shines, causing others to look to Him.

Dear God, I pray for all Your believers, that they may experience life in Your will and on Your time. Lord, open my eyes so I can trust in Your divine timeline. So I can choose Your will. Help me to not grow weary in doing good and in waiting on You! Father, write every chapter of my life, please let it **ALL** be on *YOUR TIME*.

Let us not become weary in doing good, for at the proper time we will reap a harvest if we do not give up.

Galatians 6:9 NIV

ALMIGHTY LORD

Sun shines by day
Moon and stars shine by night
Stirring up the sea with roaring waves

God, the Creator of all things, does this. His creation is part of our everyday lives. We are not in awe of this because we experience creation every day.

What if the sun stopped shining by day or the moon and stars disappeared at night? Would we stop to question?

His power is showcased every day. What is it that is too great for God?

There is so much order and beauty showcased in Your creation. Please open my eyes and help me see all the wonders around me. These things, the lovely things in Your creation, all point to the *ALMIGHTY LORD.*

This is what the LORD says, he who appoints the sun to shine by day, who decrees the moon and stars to shine by night, who stirs up the sea so that its waves roar—the LORD Almighty is his name.

Jeremiah 31:35 NIV

GREAT ARE YOU

You see all things. Do all things make You smile?

I would imagine there are things I do that hurt Your heart because of the hurt I bring upon myself or others.

Know My goodness

God's goodness is peace that transcends.
When we self-destruct out of fear or lack,
when we hurt others or ourselves, we can go
before God and He will give us peace.

God, why do I see Your goodness more on some days and not as much on others?

How much of your day are you looking to Me?
Asking Me? Coming to Me?

Dear Lord, mighty are Your deeds and great are Your purposes that lay over the world. Your eyes see it all. For the faithful ones, Father, the ones who kept pushing the plow, mighty are the winds coming towards them. Strong winds to lift them up. Under their wings, You will command the winds to **GO!** Up, up, and away! And those conducting evil, in time it shall catch up and then all shall be exposed! Oh,
GREAT ARE YOU.

Great are your purposes and mighty are your deeds. Your eyes are open to
the ways of all mankind; you reward each person according to their conduct
and as their deeds deserve.

Jeremiah 32:19 NIV

FIND ME

Vendy, I want My people to ask
I want My believers to pray to Me and come to Me
I want them to believe that I will give to them
I want them to know I'm always here,
all they have to do is knock

Yes, Lord, but at times seeking You can be hard. How do we seek You more fully?

When the desire to know Me is planted in one's heart,
My Spirit will lead the way
I will place events and people to lead them
But to seek Me is a choice and it requires belief

Belief: Acceptance that a statement is true or that something exists.

In order to seek You more fully, I must first believe You exist?

Yes

Seek and you will find. He is waiting!

Dear Lord, help us seek, believe, and find You. 🙏 Father, it is Your
desire to open the door to all. You have a table of plenty, but we
MUST believe and we **MUST** seek. Lord, I know that when
I find You, I
FIND ME.

Ask and it will be given to you; seek and you will
find; knock and the door will be opened to you.

Matthew 7:7 NIV

WRITE YOUR HEART

I am always amazed by the ways You are able to comfort me. I am always amazed by the ways You are able to love me. I am always amazed by the ways You guide me. I am always amazed by how You work things out for the best. I am always amazed by how You surprise me with plans I could have never imagined for myself. People and things I would have never dreamed of . . .

God shows us how to love. He writes cares on our hearts. He walks us through challenges and holds our hands every step of the way.

God holds the keys to great, unsearchable things . . . Things we do not know.

Dear Lord, Your ways are so much higher than mine. Your plans are so divine. I just want my entire life to be Yours. I want You to orchestrate all cares and loves in my life and on my heart. Please lead me and help me trust You, Lord. I crave heaven's will and not my own. I know how great the will from above is. Please, God, may Your will be done in our hearts as it is in heaven. Lord, on me and in me, use my life and
WRITE YOUR HEART.

This is what the LORD says, he who made the earth, the LORD who formed it and established it—the LORD is his name: "Call to me and I will answer you and tell you great and unsearchable things you do not know."

Jeremiah 33:2-3 NIV

✴ *PEACE FROM ME* ✴

Worry: Give way to anxiety or unease; allow one's mind
to dwell on difficulty or troubles.

Let your request be known to God earnestly and humbly.

Vendy, I don't like it when My children worry
Because it's a choice
for them to worry and not trust Me
And if they worry . . . it's a process only they can stop
It's part of free will and no matter how many times
I comfort them
If they allow their minds to dwell on difficulty
rather than trusting Me
It presents a challenge
many of My children face daily

How do I worry less?

More trust and belief in My goodness
More surrender to Me

Supplication: The action of asking or begging for
something earnestly or humbly.

God, You don't want me to be anxious about anything. Anything, a.k.a. all things. I should bring everything (not some things, but everything) to You in prayer with seriousness and humility.

Dear God, please help me do this. Through prayer and petition, I will practice trusting You. The more trust I have in You, the more peace I have. I will practice this daily to combat the worry that fills my mind and heart. I crave peace from You and not peace that this world offers—not
PEACE FROM ME.

> Do not be anxious about anything, but in everything by prayer and supplication with thanksgiving let your requests be made known to God. And the peace of God, which surpasses all understanding, will guard your hearts and your minds in Christ Jesus.
>
> **Philippians 4:6-7 ESV**

RENOWNED JOYS

I created this world 🌑 with all its beauty
to be enjoyed by My creation
I created relationships, families, sunsets, kisses, hugs, lattes,
puppies, palm trees, blue skies, art, food,
and the ocean waves 〰 all to be enjoyed
I created intimacy, in many different forms,
all to be enjoyed
I placed My people on earth to enjoy
all the goodness from above
So please enjoy today.
The big things and the little things
Please enjoy all I have blessed you with today
because you do not know what tomorrow holds
Only I do
And please move throughout your day knowing
how much I love you
And how much pleasure I receive when my creation smiles,
laughs, and experiences the joys
I created in the ways I intended

God receives pleasure when we smile, laugh,
and experience the joys He created in the
ways He intended.

Dear God, thank You for my peaceful morning and the abundant prosperity You provide each and every day 🤍 , even when I am not aware. When I wake each day, after spending time with You, I find that my eyes open to the simple, but
RENOWNED JOYS.

Then this city will bring me renown, joy, praise and honor before all nations on earth that hear of all the good things I do for it; and they will be in awe and will tremble at the abundant prosperity and peace I provide for it.

Jeremiah 33:9 NIV

FOREVER

Lord, thank You for loving me and choosing me, even when I don't choose myself. When I don't act in a loving way towards myself.

Thank You for seeing me in the most loving way. For when You do, I act from a place of love.

I ask for more of You and less of me.

Dear God, thank You for a new day. Thank You for Your grace. Thank You for Your enduring love and care. I pray my eyes are open more and more so I can know, trust, and live with Your love as enough
FOREVER. 🤍

Give thanks to the LORD, for he is good.
His love endures forever.

Psalm 136:1 NIV

RENEW

Give me eyes to see like You
Give me ears to hear like You
Give me a mind to think like You
Give me a heart to understand like You

When more souls seek to be renewed by Him,
more souls will hear from Him.

Dear Lord, I know it is a process to be renewed by You. Please,
Lord, help me take every experience and lay it at Your feet so
You can guide me in a way that renews how I view all situations.
Whether I turn to the right or to the left, I always want to hear
Your voice, the voice that causes us to
RENEW.

Whether you turn to the right or to the left, your ears will
hear a voice behind you, saying, "This is the way; walk in it."

Isaiah 30:21 NIV

HEART AND MIND

Above all else, guard your heart, for everything
you do flows from it.

Proverbs 4:23 NIV

So much of my life has changed.
So much of my comforts have changed.
So much of what I know, the ways I used to think,
have changed.

When seeds of doubt, worry, or fear pop into your
mind, pray to Him, ask Him, seek Him.

I'm changing the way you see things,
the way you look at people and situations
So I can take you to new places
Change from Me is good,
I will hold your hand
and walk you through it

God's love is so gentle, but so strong. He never
stops loving—even when we stop loving Him.

Dear Lord, please take my heart and mind. Hold on to my heart,
grow it, so when I feel heavy from what I see or experience and from
my thought , I can trust it is You Who takes hold of my heart.
For only You can make something new of my
HEART AND MIND.

My son, give me your heart and let your eyes delight in my ways.

Proverbs 23:26 NIV

SPOIL ME WITH YOUR LOVE

You have made my heart so tender because You have spoiled me
with Your love. 🤍 I need much of Your strength. I cling to You.

I know, I feel in my bones, the many great things You have planned.
Yet, excitement is not close to me.

Seek the LORD and his strength; seek his presence continually!

1 Chronicles 16:11 ESV

I long for You. Our time together is the best—where I feel safe and
rejuvenated. It's never long enough.

When we withdraw to desolate places and
pray 🙏 , He meets us there.

Dear Lord, help me take my time with You into the world and share
it with others! I am forever grateful for this space with You, this
safe space I have created. Our time, our sweet time together,
Lord, is where You
SPOIL ME WITH YOUR LOVE.

On my bed I remember you; I think of you through the watches
of the night. Because you are my help, I sing in the shadow
of your wings. I cling to you; your right hand upholds me.

Psalm 63:6-8 NIV

WRITE TO ME

God, I feel so much better when I write to You. I feel so much peace and gain so much clarity. When I am confused or in need of Your guidance, I can always flip back to how I was feeling and read what I wrote and what You told me.

Why did You choose the Bible, Scripture, writings to communicate to us? There must be something special about writing our thoughts and feelings. Reading words. Having something, some form of truth to hold on to . . .

God's words, instructions, and promises in
His writings do not change.

I communicate with My people in many ways:
early morning sunsets, birds chirping, waves crashing,
the sound of palm trees hugging in the wind,
but My words do not change
My words are a foundation they can stand on
My words are truth that will guide them.
My words will comfort them
My words, unlike human words, do not fail

What did He tell you today? What do His words say?

Dear Lord, I thank You for Your words today. They have given light to my life and understanding to my simple ways of thinking. I have reached a place in my faith where I find much delight in the unfolding of Your words in my life. It is almost always the highlight of each day! My God, I hear from You—I know I do! When I write all You tell me, I date it, so that when it comes to pass, I can point my family and friends to the heavens! He is real, oh so real, just look at the ways He moves in me. Oh, my God, please always

WRITE TO ME!

> The unfolding of your words gives light;
> it gives understanding to the simple.

Psalm 119:130 NIV

I CHOOSE YOU

It's My faithfulness.

Not what you say or don't say
Not what you do or don't do
Not how hard you work
Not how well you love
Not how . . .

It's My faithfulness.

The fruit and blessings of God's Spirit, the goodness He pours down and freely gives, is not based on how well we do anything.

If you are like me and get overwhelmed easily by evaluating how well or how much you do, you will tire yourself.

God chooses us every day. Imagine what our lives would look like if we chose Him every day.

He expects nothing in return but for us to love Him. He will do the rest; it is nothing you do.

We are afflicted in every way, but not crushed;
perplexed, but not driven to despair.

2 Corinthians 4:8 ESV

What are some ways we can choose God today?

Dear Father, free me. Free me of the pain that flows from the world, the weight of not always choosing the right thing. Help me see and believe that it is You moving through me, it is You working through me. I pray for more self-control and discernment. I pray for more courage to speak up and forgive. I pray for freedom in all areas and peace of mind that comes from walking in Your will. Oh, my God, *I CHOOSE YOU.*

And we impart this in words not taught by human wisdom but taught by the Spirit, interpreting spiritual truths to those who are spiritual.

1 Corinthians 2:13 ESV

SEPTEMBER

CHECK-INS

Why do I find that the more I run to God, the more I need to check in
with Him? I crave it.

I imagine God in heaven, looking down at all of His
creation. It makes Him happy to see us live. To watch us as we
go through life. He enjoys watching us, His innocent creation,
navigating the many turns in life.

I enjoy checking in with God as often
as I do because His love is so pure.
His guidance from above is honest
and truthful. We can be the most
vulnerable with God.

Dear Lord, no matter how many times You give me the same answer,
I crave my check-ins with You. *Just trust Me, sweet V.*
Search me, Lord, test my heart, my many anxious thoughts, and the
offensive ways in me, and rid me of them! Do what only You can do
and lead me in the way of everlasting peace. I pray for
more souls to crave with You these
CHECK-INS.

Search me, God, and know my heart; test me and know my anxious
thoughts. See if there is any offensive way in me, and lead me in
the way everlasting.

Psalm 139:23-24 NIV

ENRICHED IN EVERY WAY

I am there
When you feel alone and afraid,
I am there
When you feel strong and encouraged,
I am there
In every way, shape, and form,
enjoy this season because
there is never any going back

As you go through life,
you will lose people, people will find you,
and relationships will change
This is all healthy
and part of the waves 🐠 of life

Some seasons of life
you will have more to give to Me
than others

As long as God comes first in our hearts
and minds, we will always have true peace
and joy. We will always be able to give.

Dear Lord, please open my eyes so I can be grateful and aware of all You did and continue to do in my life. Help me care for those in my life who need it the most. For the blessings from You have always allowed me to give of the many resources I have. The abundant love, time, energy, grace, forgiveness, finances, and so on. I know it is You behind all this giving. Your generosity to me is what makes me *ENRICHED IN EVERY WAY.*

You will be enriched in every way so that you can be generous on every occasion, and through us your generosity will result in thanksgiving to God.

2 Corinthians 9:11 NIV

ACCORDING TO HIS PURPOSE

Why is it God? You have blessed me with everything I need to
not only survive, but thrive, and yet this world 🌍 . . . I just do not
belong! By the power of Your hand, You shape our hearts oh
so differently.

To all those who love Him and are called to His
purpose . . . keep going, for you are not alone!

The long, lonely nights. The tiring seasons. The unseen sacrifice.
The seen sacrifice. The pain-filled eyes.
Others' disbelief. **KEEP GOING!**

He has a mighty plan, but it will be only by His hand!

Why? Why would one want to put all their
eggs in one basket? 🐓

God works all things together for the good of those
who are called according to His purpose.

Dear Lord, help us see Your protection and place our trust in You.
All our cares and hopes in You. All our love in You. All our joy in
You. For I know You work everything out for the good, for those
people who are called to Your purpose. I am not a minister
by any means, just a soul called
ACCORDING TO HIS PURPOSE.

And we know that in all things God works for the good of those
who love him, who have been called according to his purpose.

Romans 8:28 NIV

PROTECTION FROM ABOVE

God appoints His angels in heaven to take care of us;
He appoints powerful angels to watch our steps.

> For he will command his angels concerning
> you to guard you in all your ways.
>
> **Psalm 91:11 NIV**

Soooo these powerful angels watch over all those who dwell close to
the Lord to guard us in not just **SOME** of our ways or **SOME** areas,
but **ALL** our ways, and **ALL** areas of our lives.

> The powers above watch over God's children,
> innocent lambs among wolves.
>
> Now go, and remember that I am sending
> you out as lambs among wolves.
>
> **Luke 10:3 NLT**

If you believe you are protected in the highest form from powers
above, then you will be called and appointed to those who need it the
most. As a result, don't be surprised if the Lord places kingdoms of
the world 🌍 and powers from above at
your fingertips.

Dear Lord, help me to do for You whatever You ask of me. Lord,
help me trust. I will go where You want me to go, I will love who
You want me to love. Please, Lord, remove fear and grow my trust.
All I need is more trust in You and I promise I will serve

whoever it is You want me to serve. Lord, it is You I look to and You Who appoints the powerful angels to look after me! It is Your mighty *PROTECTION FROM ABOVE.*

> Take him and look after him; don't harm him
> but do for him whatever he asks.

Jeremiah 39:12 NIV

LOVERS OF GOD

Lovers of pleasure rather than lovers of God; what does that
look like?

I think it means I trust more in my desires than God.

I think it means I trust more in my thoughts than God.

I think it means I trust more in the ways of the world
rather than letting the most powerful Spirit lead and
be my guide.

His Holy Spirit fills this world with more
lovers of God.

What does that look like?

You may proclaim the excellencies of Him who called
you out of darkness into His marvelous light.

1 Peter 2:9 NASB

Dear Lord, I know it is You Who holds my right hand; You hold
on to it so tightly and You guide me. However, I like to jump
ahead! I know, in a way that shows great attention to detail, You are
meticulously writing every chapter of my life. Yet, I so want to jump
ahead at times! I want to know what's next. I want to know why now
rather than patiently waiting and trusting in You as You divinely

unfold my path. I pray for more lovers of God and less lovers of pleasure to fill this earth. I pray for less fear and more wisdom from above 🙏 to direct our steps! Father, You are forever at my side, You are my never-ending guide. Oh, Lord, I pray for more

LOVERS OF GOD!

For I, the Lord your God, hold your right hand; it is I who say to you, "Fear not, I am the one who helps you."

Isaiah 41:13 ESV

I WILL DO ALL THAT I PLEASE

My goodness is all around you
I need you to stop being fearful and trust
Trust the blessing and fruit of your life
Trust I am here
In the midst
Trust I am going before you
Trust I whisper truth to others on your behalf
Trust I am making the way
Trust when you don't understand

I am not asking you
to trust in anything but Me, sweet V
And the beauty in that is
I never fail because I am God
The beauty in that is
I always deliver far beyond
I am always on time.
I always lead you to more joy,
peace, love, and light
I am the way, the best possible way,
and I promise to never leave you, honey

Placing our trust in God does not always make sense
to this world, and it does not always come easy, but
when we do, we never fail. God places us on the best
possible path. One we could have never ventured
on without Him.

Dear God, please help me to trust. I have seen many wonders You
have weaved throughout my life, and I hope to see more. Please,
God, help me to trust You more and nothing else. Just You because
You are the beginning and the end, so the things You have whispered
to me were the end from the beginning and much of what is still to
come—it is so praiseworthy. I must tell the world to **WAIT** on the
Lord. Friends, family, and souls, wait on the Alpha and the Omega,
for He is for you and His purpose will stand. He will do all that
He pleases because He is God, the Creator of all,
Who said to me this morning, *Sweet V,*
I WILL DO ALL THAT I PLEASE.

I make known the end from the beginning, from ancient times,
what is still to come. I say, "My purpose will stand, and
I will do all that I please."

Isaiah 46:10 NIV

✦ *TOGETHER* ✦

What is next is beautiful, My sweet child,
and we will do it together
We will be together because you know
how much you need My guidance
Because you enjoy time with Me, sweet V

Together: In companionship or close association.

Time with God is all you need for
all that is next for you.

∽Time with Me strengthens you∽
∽Time with Me helps you see∽
∽Time with Me helps you hear∽
∽Time with Me helps you love∽
∽Time with Me helps you trust∽

Dear Lord, together we will accomplish all that is next because
I have grown oh so close to You. I sit and wait for You to tell me
when to move, where to go, how to act, and what to say. Because
You have made my mind like You, sharing love and delight for what
You love and delight in. My spirit goes before, Your Spirit goes
before . . . and does the deed, accomplishes what it needs.
Father, let us step into all that is next
TOGETHER.

Then make my joy complete by being like-minded, having
the same love, being one in spirit and of one mind.

Philippians 2:2 NIV

ORPHANS AND WIDOWS

God is close to the fatherless.

God is close to the widows.

Women and children have a special place in God's heart.
He cares a great deal for their well-being and safety.

If there is one religion you practice, let it be this:
Care for the needs of women and children, the
orphans and widows. For, in God's eyes, this is the
most pure and faultless religion.

Children are so pure and only know so much. In this world, what is
more vulnerable than a child?

Women physically tend to be weaker vessels, so when harm is
inflicted upon them physically by a stronger source, this pains God.
It is an abuse of power on His creation.

How do you keep your mind, heart, and actions from being polluted
by the ways of this world?

Finally, brothers, whatever is true, whatever is honorable,
whatever is just, whatever is pure, whatever is lovely, whatever
is commendable, if there is any excellence, if there is anything
worthy of praise, think about these things.

Philippians 4:8 ESV

Dear God, I love what You call pure and blameless in Your sight because it so happens to be another care written on my heart. My mother is a widow. My three little nieces, the ones she is raising by herself, are orphans and do not have a mother or father to look after them. Father, I have seen how You have so powerfully guarded my mother and three nieces. Although I have asked You **WHY** many times, I no longer need the answer because You are greater than the why. You, my God, are the how! May I continue to look to my mother Nicole and see that the how is You! You look after the widows and orphans with an extra eye! Today I pray for all Your children. I pray for the single mothers; I pray for children without parents. I pray for Your innocent creation. Lord, in Your eyes, there is nothing more important and pure of heart than looking after those who need it the most. Lord, in Your eyes, there is nothing more important than guarding our hearts and minds from the harshness of this world 🌍 , and one way to do this is to look after the *ORPHANS AND WIDOWS*.

Religion that God our Father accepts as pure and faultless is this:
to look after orphans and widows in their distress and
to keep oneself from being polluted by the world.

James 1:27 NIV

MY SPIRIT DWELLS

My dear daughter
My Spirit dwells in you
A vessel that carries Me
My love, My compassion,
My tender heart for people

Dwell: To live or stay as a permanent resident; reside. To live or continue in a given condition or state.

God's Spirit dwells in people.

For God's Spirit to dwell in and with us, the conditions of our bodies and minds must be pure. We will always fall short of His goodness, but when we meditate on all that is honorable, truthful, loving, and good, the conditions of our minds and bodies allow His Spirit to reside in us.

Much of our power lies in being able to dwell with God's Spirit.

What happens when His Spirit dwells with us?

We make decisions that bring more love into our lives and into the lives of others. Our vision is transformed, and we have more compassionate eyes.

Dear Lord, I know there are many areas where I fall short. I know these areas are where there is a lack of You. A sign of where I need more of Your Spirit to dwell. Please, Lord, send Your Spirit and show us the places in our lives where we need to invite You in. Please, Lord, help me in all my weakness and teach me where I need more of You. Send Your Spirit and teach me how to pray; allow us to become one so with You

MY SPIRIT DWELLS.

In the same way, the Spirit helps us in our weakness. We do not know what we ought to pray for, but the Spirit himself intercedes for us through wordless groans.

Romans 8:26 NIV

RECOGNIZABLE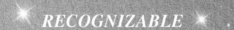

Your Spirit is recognizable in this world.

Recognize: Identify (someone or something) from having encountered them before.

What does that look like?

In this world?
In God's eyes?
In evil's eyes?
In truth's eyes?
In love's eyes?

We always have a choice in this life. To be recognized in the eyes of truth, love, and all that flows from above is a sign. To also identify evil because it's the opposite of what you identify with, is powerful. To identify evil because you've encountered it makes it recognizable.

For he chose us in him before the creation of the world
to be holy and blameless in his sight.

Ephesians 1:4 NIV

There is a divine law at work in the world with a simple spectrum:

Purity∽Sin

When we choose all that is pure and just, we become Christlike. And thanks to Jesus, we have an option to be recognized by all that flows from above. 🙏

Dear Lord, my sweet Father in heaven, I want to be recognized by You. I want a spirit that shines. That brings glory to You. I want others to be able to see You. I want to be marked by You. For my battle is never with other humans, never with flesh and blood, but against the ruling authorities, the powers of darkness that operate in the spiritual word. I know this sounds crazy to people who do not know You. Let me just say, if only you knew, experienced or tasted the goodness of God like I have, you would know that the forces of evil at play in our day-to-day could **NEVER** be of and from Him. Ever. You would know that without His light, the darkness of night would consume you. You would know that the dark forces do not sleep, and so God never stops working on your behalf. You would know that the meanness in another, the evildoing in another, is not truly them but the dwelling of recognized evil that has taken root in them. I know this because I am a soul who has journeyed through much darkness. I come to testify of the power and glory that lives in the light! The Lamb of the world has won, and evil has no claim on me, but it does on some I love . . . so, Father, I pray pray pray in Your eyes always may I be
RECOGNIZABLE.

For our struggle is not against flesh and blood, but against the
rulers, against the authorities, against the powers of this dark world
and against the spiritual forces of evil in the heavenly realms.

Ephesians 6:12 NIV

DESIRES OF ONE

You will seek me and find me when you seek me
with all your heart.

Jeremiah 29:13 NIV

Lord, by Your hand You have transformed the shape of
my heart. 🤍 You have formed me into a new creation.

One that sees less as more
One that loves honesty and simplicity
One that prefers few rather than many
One that needs much rest
and time with You alone
One that desires only One

One that hopes, but only with You
One that gives, but only with You
One that opens up, but only with You
One that forgives, but only with You

You gave me vision when I was blind
You are my strength, my confidence, my identity
Your love grows   me to new heights
Your steadiness grounds me
Your humility purifies me
May I always be amazed by Your love
Your sweet, tender love

May You always be my everything
May You always be my truth,
my light, my hope, my joy
My One

Peace will come when more souls make
Him their number one.

Dear Lord, You have heard my every cry. You were near
and saved me. When I wanted to stay and lay, You told me
to **GET UP** and stand because I was chosen by You. You
told me I would water many souls when I had no more water left
in me. You told me I would be a light when I had no light in me.
You said I would be powerful when I was weak. You said I would
feed many when I could not eat! You carried me when I could not
walk and loved me when I did not have any love left in me. So how
could I want anything more than You? You Who is so good to me.
You Who gave me hope when I had none. You Who is with me in
the morning and the evening, in my coming and my going. It is You
Who I belong to and promise to be faithful to! I am for You, and if
You do not answer another prayer of mine, if this is the only request
I ever send up, let it be my desire for the One and Only You. You
Who grew my heart and formed my desires after You.
Now the world will read and see the
DESIRES OF ONE.

The LORD is near to all who call on him, to all who call on him in
truth. He fulfills the desires of those who fear him; he hears their
cry and saves them.

Psalm 145:18-19 NIV

NEVER LET GO

You have divine permission
Consent to enjoy this beautiful life
I am creating for you
Filled with wonder and miracles

Trust in the LORD with all your heart, and do not
lean on your own understanding. In all your ways
acknowledge him, and he will make straight
your paths.

Proverbs 3:5-6 ESV

A life that was originally intended for My creation:
One where they enjoy the simple
and big things equally, so they have joy every day
One where they can see and feel Me in their every day
One where My Spirit is their ultimate guide
One where they always find comfort in Me
A life where a simple thought from the heart
becomes a reality

The key to this life is choosing God each day
and placing Him at the center daily.

I am the all-powerful God Whose love knows no limits
Like a warm blanket, My love will guard you
from the harshest environments
And keep you warm on the coldest of nights
My blanket will always be there for you to pick up
When you choose Me, I will write every chapter
I will never let go of the pen ✒

Dear God, there is too much favor for me to speak of. Every good and perfect thing I have in my life is from and of You. My favorite part: You are consistent and will always be there to bless me. Bless me with more of You! Your Spirit, quiet time, love, hope, grace, and just what I need. Should I get busy and enter a season when I work from my own strength like I tend to do, then just dim the lights and bring me back to You. For with You, nothing can come against me that will prosper, but rather You cause it to make me prosper! Oh, my God, never leave me, please
NEVER LET GO.

Every good gift and every perfect gift is from above,
coming down from the Father of lights, with whom
there is no variation or shadow due to change.

James 1:17 ESV

OPEN EYES

The LORD is good to all, and his mercy is over all that he has made.

Psalm 145:9 ESV

How do I open My creation's eyes?
I make them aware of all I do for them
Of the many ways
I string their lives together for the good
Of the many ways I show compassion
Of the many ways they experience love

Invite Him in and hand it to Him.

Good: Benefit or advantage to someone or something.

Compassion: Concern for the sufferings or misfortunes of others.

Love: Deep affection.

Dear Lord, thank You for creating a life full of Your goodness, never-ending compassion, and complete love. I pray for more eyes to be opened to realize it is You Who is for them and working all things together for their good. May more souls invite You into their pain, for it is those You love and choose that You work it all together for their good. Please, Father, *OPEN EYES.*

And we know that for those who love God all things work together for good, for those who are called according to his purpose.

Romans 8:28 ESV

LOST SOULS

Vendy, pray for those in your life who need it the most

Why?

Because that is the way My kingdom works,
that is the design I have put in place

Prayers that go up offer direct protection.
Prayers that go up replace worry.
Prayers that go up fight the
will of the adversary.

Soul: Emotional or intellectual energy.

Lost souls do not know My love
They do not experience the abundance of My fruits:
Peace, love, joy, patience, kindness, goodness, gentleness,
faithfulness, and self-control
They walk this world 🌐 and experience much pain
Pain that needs deep emotional and physical healing

How do we help these souls?

Prayer with a truthful heart is powerful and effective

Prayer: Integration with God; a request for help or expression
of thanks addressed to God; an earnest hope or wish.

Dear Father, I pray for the lost souls. I pray for the lost
souls whose families long to have them close. I pray for the lost
souls that do not know Your love and choose choose choose pain.
I pray for one lost soul specifically today, my sister. I lift her up to
You. The chains of darkness have their hold on her. Her life has been
filled with suffering that Your hand has no part of. Suffering that
hurts Your eyes and is too great for me to speak. God, I know there
are more souls out there like my sister who just need You so they can
be free of the lies that enter their minds. Oh, Lord, many days pass
and I do not pray for her because she is removed in many ways. Her
ways that cause her to stray have hurt me and those I love the most;
I have learned to hand it over to You. But then there are days, days I
wake and feel something horrible is going to happen to her because
of the sad way she lives. She is the most lost soul I know and needs
You, Lord, so hear me! Hear my prayers, Lord, and make them
powerful and effective to Your ears. Allow them to command armies
of Your angels to fight the demons that surround her. Please, Lord,
save her and bring her back home because You can. Only You, Lord,
have the power to. Stop the hurting, mourning heart of my mother
and bring her back. God, I pray for all the
LOST SOULS.

Therefore confess your sins to each other and pray for each other
so that you may be healed. The prayer of a righteous person
is powerful and effective.

James 5:16 NIV

OCTOBER

TRUST IN MY

Power: Ability to do something with quality.

Wisdom: Good judgment, experience, knowledge.

Understanding: Sympathetic awareness or tolerance.

Do we trust God's power? Do we trust God's
wisdom? Do we trust God's understanding?

Peace: Freedom from disturbance; tranquility or
mental calm; serenity.

My flesh limits me. My paradigm is not from above,
so I can only know so much. Because of this, I can
never trust fully in my own wisdom, power,
and understandings.

Dear God, I pray for peace. Please freely give Your people peace.
Peace that flows from trusting in You. Trusting in Your power,
wisdom, and understanding. My God, You created the earth by Your
power and founded the world by Your wisdom. You stretched out the
heavens with Your understanding. What is it You cannot do? What is
it You would like me to trust in? You name it, I am here and
will be here all morning!
TRUST IN MY . . .?

He made the earth by his power; he founded the world by his wisdom
and stretched out the heavens by his understanding.

Jeremiah 51:15 NIV

CARES

How do you view yourself? A scale with worldly measurements
destroys your confidence.

We as humans have cares, many cares placed
on our hearts. There is power in
acknowledging these cares—freedom even.

The world can make us feel as though our cares create weakness
in our lives.

Many cares create depth, truth, beauty, and
fulfillment in your life.

God has placed many joys in my life. Some complex, some simple.
Why do I find comfort hiding behind the simple joys?

Spending more time with the Creator of all
things washes away the world's impressions
and scars that live on our hearts.

Dear Lord, I pray for more time with You. Spending time with
You builds my confidence in all areas and exposes the truths
You have placed on my heart. This transforms my soul and
strengthens my humanity. Oh, how You have planted dreams that
stem from my many
CARES . . .

A dream comes when there are many cares.

Ecclesiastes 5:3 NIV

WORTHY

*None of My children are truly worthy of My love,
yet they receive it fully
This is part of My goodness, My sovereignty
So love people, even if you feel they do not deserve your love at
all times, sweet V*

Do everything without grumbling or arguing, so that you
may become blameless and pure, "children of God without fault
in a warped and crooked generation." Then you will shine among
them like stars in the sky as you hold firmly to the word of life.

Philippians 2:14-16 NIV

God enjoys when we . . .

Cling to Him. Desire to hear from Him.

Why?

Quality time and communication (listening and talking) are part
of any relationship. When you are in relationship with people, you
desire to spend time with them. You simply enjoy it!

The more time we spend with God,
the deeper our love grows.

No human can do what God can do for you.

No human can ever love you the way God can love you.

To experience our Creator's love is a gift. His love
protects our lives and creates purity, which is
also a gift. A gift that points to above. 🖤

Dear Lord, I am not worthy of Your love, but I am grateful. You have
given me a pure heart and steadfast spirit! I pray more souls learn to
cling to You in the good and bad. When it is sunny and dark, in the
winter, fall, spring, and summer! I pray more souls desire to hear
from You. I know they do, they just need Your help getting there,
and sometimes it takes a bending of both knees. Worthy of Your love
I am not, but Your praise I will sing for all You have done for me.
It will forever be
WORTHY.

Create in me a pure heart, O God, and renew
a steadfast spirit within me.

Psalm 51:10 NIV

WAYS OF THE LORD

I want for My children . . .
I want nothing more than for My children
to be blameless
My sweet daughter

Why?

So they can ride every wave with ease
So they can do all things through Me

How do we become blameless?

You trust in Me with all your
heart, mind, body, and soul
You trust in My ways

Trust in the LORD with all your heart and
lean not on your own understanding.

Proverbs 3:5 NIV

The desires of your heart, He knows. He wrote
them, so hurry up and bend a knee. Trust in
your Creator. Trust in the Lord and He will bring
about all that needs to be.

Dear Lord, I pray for Your people everywhere. That our
eyes be open to **ALL** Your truths in Your words. May Your Spirit
come alongside us and guide us to lead blameless lives.

Lives free of shame, fear, and evil. Free us from temptation and grant us freedom from evil. May we learn to walk in the *WAYS OF THE LORD.*

Blessed are those whose ways are blameless,
who walk according to the law of the LORD.

Psalm 119:1 NIV

THREE POWERS

You, Lord, are forgiving and good, abounding in
love to all who call to you.

Psalm 86:5 NIV

Why, Lord, is a relationship with You so powerful?

Why, Lord, do I feel so safe with You?

Why, Lord, do I crave You?

∽You are honest∽
∽Your love is consistent∽
∽You protect my mind, heart, soul, and body∽

Honesty, love, and protection is a powerful
combination in any relationship.

Dear Lord, thank You for filling me. Your honesty, love, and
protection have taught me so much. Help me follow Your command
and love each person as You have loved me. For this is a desire of
Your heart, a desire for Your people to experience and to see the
THREE POWERS.

My command is this: Love each
other as I have loved you.

John 15:12 NIV

BOOK OF LIFE

Do whatever You have to do to me, Lord. Do what only You can do.
Make me a vessel.

Your heart, your life,
you, My creation, are enough
Pick up and carry My fire.
Hold it close and I will keep it burning
Because I am the fuel,
your flame will never go out
Winds and consuming waters
have no power over My flames
It's My mighty Spirit that keeps
these eternal flames going

Please, just hold it close
My fire will guide you,
it will give you new power
and grant new freedom to you
And all who dwell close

Don't you know that you yourselves are God's temple and
that God's Spirit dwells in your midst?

1 Corinthians 3:16 NIV

His ever-burning flame will guide you.

Each one's work will become manifest, for the Day will disclose
it, because it will be revealed by fire, and the fire will test what
sort of work each one has done.

1 Corinthians 3:13 ESV

Thank You for today. Thank You for all You have done and continue to do. 🙏 My sweet Father, You are breaking new ground. Write the book of my life. Please, help me give my life, all of myself, to You. Let each page burn with Your glory. 🔥 I pray You write my *BOOK OF LIFE.*

For our God is a consuming fire.

Hebrews 12:29 NIV

OUR HEARTS ADORE

Orphans now have a home
Hopeless have found a home

∽All You Have Done∽

The sun did rise on my darkest nights
You did lift my weary head
You turned my weakness into strength

Brothers and sisters, we do not want you to be uninformed
about those who sleep in death, so that you do not grieve
like the rest of mankind, who have no hope.

1 Thessalonians 4:13 NIV

God, my heart truly adores You because I've experienced much of
Your goodness. Your great mercy and love, which showed up when
I needed it the most. On the coldest of nights.

I see visions of brokenness. A globe filled with people everywhere
crawling through life, fighting. Single mothers, exhausted and alone;
children who do not know the love of a mother or a father; verbal
and physical abuse of the weak; death and loss of love; low self-
esteem in humans; absence of respect; and people with little hope
because of injustice in every area.

Lord, so many weary heads. So much pain and suffering.

∽All You've Done∽Our Hearts Adore∽
∽Our Affection∽Our Devotion∽

Adore: Love and respect deeply, worship, venerate, to speak and pray to.

Oh, hopeless soul, turn to the Lord! Turn to the Lord for Your hearts to adore. 🙏

Dear Lord, my heart so greatly adores You. Oh, how I love You. 🕊️ Your love has stayed the same while old things have passed away. I pray for all who do not know You, all who go through life fighting, making a way on their own strength. Because of Jesus, we can live in the midst of injustice, great pain, and endless suffering and bring love and light with us. We can be new. We can have hope and bring love to dark places. Jesus, You gave breath to death and made a way when there was no way. You, Prince of Peace,
OUR HEARTS ADORE.

For to us a child is born, to us a son is given, and the government will be on his shoulders. And he will be called Wonderful Counselor, Mighty God, Everlasting Father, Prince of Peace.

Isaiah 9:6 NIV

SHELTER OF THE MOST HIGH

Search my heart, Lord. Tell me what causes me to stumble.
What hurts You?

Your lack of trust, Vendy
I speak to your heart,
I give you signs for what is just around the corner
I strategically hold your life in My hands
and it pains Me when you don't trust
As a result, your desires get twisted, you grow impatient
Your thoughts are full of doubt
regarding My goodness in your life . . .
When I, My sweet daughter,
am always the One Who blesses you
I delight in being able to bless My children
I have designed life for My creation to always be unpredictable
That way they learn to lean on Me and choose Me
Your life, all of my creation's lives, will always be this;
You will never truly know what tomorrow will bring,
but with Me as your guide
You will have peace
and the more you learn to trust and rely on Me
The better because I can protect you
from worry and stress . . . from exhaustion
Just continue to look to Me

Continue to look to Him daily! May His presence go before You, and beside You, all around You.
He is with You!

When times are good, be happy; but when times are bad, consider this: God has made the one as well as the other. Therefore, no one can discover anything about their future.

Ecclesiastes 7:14 NIV

How do I keep You first?

You choose Me in little ways

How do I know what way is Your way?

Whatever is true, whatever is noble, whatever is right, whatever is pure, whatever is lovely, whatever is admirable—if anything is excellent or praiseworthy—think about such things.

Philippians 4:8 NIV

Dear Lord, You know the exact recipe for my life. You know every ingredient, You know how much to add, what to remove, and how to mix it in at just the right temperature so I become the best version of myself. You know our lives' events are all part of a master recipe. Please, Lord, continue to craft the ultimate recipe, bringing peace and prosperity so we turn out exactly the way You have planned, by Your hand, in the
SHELTER OF THE MOST HIGH.

My son, do not forget my teaching, but keep my commands in your heart, for they will prolong your life many years and bring you peace and prosperity.

Proverbs 3:1-2 NIV

AS DREAMERS DO

With Him, anything your heart desires will come to you. No request is too extreme for the Creator of all things! He is the Creator of all the stars, of all that is true and beautiful. ⭐

If His love is at the center of your dream, then
God will see it through. Ask whatever you
wish, and if it is of His will, it will be
done for you.

And this is the confidence that we have toward him, that
if we ask anything according to his will he hears us.

1 John 5:14 ESV

No request to Me is too extreme
Oh, if only My creation knew
the dreams I have for them
The beautiful plans, the magic, and the wonder
The details rest in My hand and
the timeline is divine
I have the power to see it all through . . .
For all to come true in a way so mighty
So well-orchestrated,
no eye has seen, no ear has heard

Keep faith, hold it close to you heart 🤍
and pray to me
Anything your heart desires will come
to you through Me

Dear Lord, I have asked much of You. I pray often to You.
I pray for my selfish needs and desires. I pray for those I
love—my family and my friends. I pray for those in need, but,
Father, I rarely pray for You. So today I ask, What is it You wish?
And whatever that may be, Lord, I pray for it to exist. Father, You
have created me so uniquely, You have created me to dream. Which
means, since I am created in Your image, You dream! Lord, tell me
Your dreams and use me! I want to be part of Your ministry. The
ministry teamed with angels. Lord, I am like You,
so keep me dreaming
AS DREAMERS DO.

If you abide in me, and my words abide in you, ask
whatever you wish, and it will be done for you.

John 15:7 ESV

HOLD ME TIGHT

I want You to hold me tight, Lord, so I only see what You want
me to see. 99 I only hear what You want me to hear.
I only go where You want me to go.

My dear God, please hold me tight.

Tell me when to open. Tell me when to close. Show me how to love.
Paint me a picture and fill it with details, details from above I can
hold on to, I can hope for. Paint me a picture filled with Your colors,
laced with justice and love.

Ask and seek Him so you may learn to understand
His ways more and more each day.

God is the Creator of steadfast love, justice, and
righteousness. His kindness transforms the way
we view ourselves, our lives, and others. His
kindness changes the way we treat others.

Dear Lord, I pray we grow to understand You more and learn to
know You. May we learn Your ways. The ways from above.
May these ways create change and mighty shifts. Shifts in high
schools, universities, corporations, and homes! Father, I ask that
more people come to You with their pain, that they give You time to
transform them. Then, may they step back into the world once

Your healing is complete and give of the great understanding they gained. For this understanding allows me to allow You to *HOLD ME TIGHT.*

That he understands and knows me, that I am the LORD who practice
steadfast love, justice, and righteousness in the earth; for in these things
I delight, says the LORD.

Jeremiah 9:24 RSV

HOLY MOMENTS

Take me back to where we started.

Help me to just want You.

My soul clings to You; You have been my help.

And rising very early in the morning, while it was still dark, he
departed and went out to a desolate place, and there he prayed.

Mark 1:35 ESV

Why nothing else? Because You, Lord, are all I need. And when I
begin to think I need more, my heart and mind get weighed down. I
am removed from Your presence. I fail to trust You. Lord, You have
brought me so far. I just want to be caught up in Your presence. It's
these holy moments that light my life and strengthen me.

Mighty things happen when we desire
Him most. He begins to pave
His way.

Dear Lord, I pray we learn to want You more than anything You
could ever do. Help us open up our hearts to You. May You write
cares and desires on our hearts and purify our every move! 🤍
Lord, it's the holy moments in my room, with my morning matcha,
afternoon tea, and walks with the sea breeze that have gotten me
through. These holy moments will one day add up and create a
mighty movement—a mighty outpouring of Your Spirit. I can feel

it! All due to the tiny little knee that was bent to You. All due to the holy moments where You were my help. In the shadow of Your wing, I will now rise and show the world the power in
HOLY MOMENTS.

When I remember you upon my bed, and meditate on you in the watches of the night; for you have been my help, and in the shadow of your wings I will sing for joy. My soul clings to you; your right hand upholds me.

Psalm 63:6-8 ESV

SPIRIT OF THE LORD

Let Me deal with all that affects you
All the hurts of your heart
All that you do not understand
All that feels too heavy
All that is unjust
Let Me enter into these areas
of your life and take hold
So you remain steady
with peace and innocence
So you rise above and beyond

Friends, family, readers, to all with open ears: Where the Spirit of the Lord is there is freedom.

Dear Lord, my sweet Father in heaven, thank You for giving me the keys. The solutions to my frustration. My pain. My confusion. My weakness. Thank You for the fuel You provide on the days where I am running on empty. Please, Lord, I pray for more of Your Spirit to enter our lives. For more freedom. For far less stress and worry. For peace and love. For kindness and grace. For wisdom and courage. For respect and hope. For tender hearts and strong minds. For fueled bodies and restful days under the sun. I now have Your Spirit in me, so what could stop me? I pray for more souls to walk with the **SPIRIT OF THE LORD.**

Now the Lord is the Spirit, and where the Spirit of the Lord is, there is freedom.

2 Corinthians 3:17 NIV

I GIVE YOU PEACE

My sweet daughter, choose Me today
I am training you, preparing you
Choosing Me over fear and anxiety
is an everyday decision
When your walk is blameless,
there is not much the enemy has to work with.
To use against you
But the enemy will always and
can always go to the future
The unknown, to make you anxious

Placing our trust in God is an **EVERYDAY**
practice. It is designed for our benefit. Like
a muscle, the more you work it, the
stronger you become.

Trusting Me, having mighty faith, is a muscle,
and the more you use it, the stronger you grow
The less the future or anxiety can weigh on you
This is key to removing it of its power

I want My children's lives to be
in a beautiful state of bliss
Not because they do not see or hear

Or have a tender heart for
all that takes place in the world 🌍,
all the pain, but because . . .
They see Me first
They see My power
They see My greatness
All they experience that is
evil has no effect on the peaceful mind
I bless them with
On the bountiful bliss

And all they don't see is filled with trust
Trust in Me, the grand author of their life
The Creator of all that is good

God loves to give. He delights to bless
His people, but there is a muscle that
must be strong to handle all He plans
to do for you.

Dear Lord, I pray more souls practice choosing You every day in
both large and small ways. Or maybe even just small and You can do
the rest. 🤍 For the more we learn to turn to You, the more You turn
Your face to us and say,
I GIVE YOU PEACE.

The LORD bless you and keep you; the LORD make his face shine
on you and be gracious to you; the LORD turn his face toward you
and give you peace.

Numbers 6:24-26 NIV

I AM CLOSE TO YOU

Therefore, as God's chosen people, holy and dearly loved,
clothe yourselves with compassion, kindness, humility,
gentleness and patience.

Colossians 3:12 NIV

Vendy, much of your fear
stems from not believing I am close to you
Did you know . . .
As you venture throughout your day . . .
as you type and you work, as you interact
I am close to you

Why do we want to be close to God?

Because I am Truth and Love
Your heart, once it experiences
My gentle love and kind truth, adores
It needs more of this
Because My love and truth is not of this world
and I created you to be in relationship
Close relationship, with Me

Dear Lord, I pray for more of Your Spirit today and every day. More of Your Spirit, Lord, gives strength. More of Your Spirit gives us courage. And more of You creates a light yoke. More of You brings favor. More of You is rest for our souls. Lord, thank You for choosing me. Help me continue to choose You, for I want more of You. I will continue to draw near. I know, I can feel

I AM CLOSE TO YOU.

Take my yoke upon you and learn from me, for I am gentle and humble in heart, and you will find rest for your souls.

Matthew 11:29 NIV

WHAT DO YOU SEE?

I see a vast ocean 🌊 accompanied by a soft sky. I see palm trees and people riding their bikes in the early morning. I see green bundles with magenta poking out. I sit on a hill with a concrete street and see homes perched with a view of Your creation.

This is all in my backyard, all freely available once I step outside my house. Some days I see it. The beauty of a sunset walk. Some days I feel it in the wind. Other days I don't.

He opens eyes so we can see His beauty
all around us—when it's dark and
when it's sunny.

Dear God, You are all around us and with us, but setting aside time for just You grows our awareness. Grows our hearts, grows our excitement 🤍 for You. With this excitement comes all that is good! Help us meditate on Your words so You can transform us and all we see! Oh, I love all I see through this new lens! I see light win and evil flee! I see angels and mighty things! I see the good run in triumph! I see hope all around me. Only You can give this lens in a broken world. Father, ask Your people to speak. Ask them,
WHAT DO YOU SEE?

Whoever gives thought to the word will discover good.

Proverbs 16:20 ESV

NOVEMBER

WAIT FOR ME

When you trust in Me
and walk with Me,
your life operates
within My divine timeline

Wait for the Lord
Be strong
Let your heart grow courage
Wait for the Lord

For there is a time and a way for everything,
although man's trouble lies heavy on him.

Ecclesiastes 8:6 ESV

God develops us to the point of readiness.

There is always something new I am setting my eyes on. My mind gets filled and consumed. The waters are still and I'm ready for them to move. The waves crash and I'm ready for them to be still. Help me, God, to wait on You. The waiting can be hard, but You grant contentment in the midst of it. When I wait for You, I am ripe.

Contentment and gratitude in the midst of
waiting leads to a peaceful life. One full
of change, growth, and beauty. Blessings
that come and go. Blessings that stay forever.

Dear God, please teach me how to wait on Your timeline
with peace and joy. Teach me Your ways. Show me how!
I want to be ripe for Your harvest. Lord, help me wait for You. Help
me trust in You. When I do this, You heal me and strengthen me. You
open my eyes to what I do not see. You help me reach new heights.
My God, I love the ways You speak to me, I love it when You say,

Sweet V, it's already done. Just
WAIT FOR ME.

Wait for the LORD; be strong, and let your
heart take courage; wait for the LORD!

Psalm 27:14 ESV

LIFE WITH YOU

You make our lives sweet, sweet as honeycomb 🍯
You revive our souls

His testimonies make wise the simple.
His precepts cause rejoicing of the heart.
His commands are pure, enlightening
our eyes.

Dear Lord, help us desire You more. More than anything. You open our eyes to simple truths that bring peace. You overpower negative emotions and replace them with comfort. Your law, Your ways keep me safe and enlighten my eyes. There is nothing more sweet, powerful, and miraculous than a
LIFE WITH YOU.

Its rising is from the end of the heavens, and its circuit to the end of them, and there is nothing hidden from its heat. The law of the Lord is perfect, reviving the soul; the testimony of the Lord is sure, making wise the simple; the precepts of the Lord are right, rejoicing the heart; the commandment of the Lord is pure, enlightening the eyes; the fear of the Lord is clean, enduring forever; the rules of the Lord are true, and righteous altogether. More to be desired are they than gold, even much fine gold; sweeter also than honey and drippings of the honeycomb.

Psalm 19:6-10 ESV

MY PROMISES

Don't forget My promises,
My dear daughter

When we remember His promises, we have
greater hope and excitement.

The LORD himself goes before you and will be with you;
he will never leave you nor forsake you. Do not be
afraid; do not be discouraged."

Deuteronomy 31:8 NIV

I have told you these things, so that in me you may
have peace. In this world you will have trouble.
But take heart! I have overcome the world.

John 16:33 NIV

I will instruct you and teach you in the way you
should go; I will counsel you with my loving
eye on you.

Psalm 32:8 NIV

Come to me, all you who are weary and burdened,
and I will give you rest. Take my yoke upon you
and learn from me, for I am gentle and humble
in heart, and you will find rest for your souls.

Matthew 11:28-29 NIV

The LORD makes firm the steps of the one who
delights in him; though he may stumble, he
will not fall, for the LORD upholds him
with his hand.

Psalm 37:23-24 NIV

"For I know the plans I have for you," declares the
LORD, "plans to prosper you and not to harm
you, plans to give you hope and a future."

Jeremiah 29:11 NIV

And we know that in all things God works
for the good of those who love him, who
have been called according to his purpose.

Romans 8:28 NIV

Dear Lord, my sweet Father in heaven, help me to be still. Help me listen to Your gentle Spirit so You can do the rest. My soul desires Your promises. 🙏 My God, as I write to You today, I understand the power of Your words when You say to us, "Be still." When we are still, we create space for You to move on our behalf. When You direct us to be still, it means You are up to something in our lives. God, I have seen You fight my battles and move on my behalf. This usually only happens when I am still. We need only to be still to see Your mighty plans for our lives unfold. Oh, I can't wait to see the beautiful things You have spoken over me. I just can't wait to see

MY PROMISES!

The LORD will fight for you;
you need only to be still.

Exodus 14:14 NIV

MY WIND

Then a wind from the LORD sprang up.

Numbers 11:31 ESV

Do you see how powerful the wind is? Wind uproots trees. Wind shakes creations made by man. Wind directs the sea.

Wind is invisible. You do not know which way it will move or how. The human eye cannot see the wind, but we can feel and hear it.

For he commanded and raised the stormy
wind, which lifted up the waves of the sea.

Psalm 107:25 ESV

When it's windy out, all people know. They may not be able to see it, but they can hear and feel it. They see the effects of the wind.

A move of God, like moves of the
wind, is recognizable by all.

And suddenly there came from heaven a sound
like a mighty rushing wind, and it filled the
entire house where they were sitting.

Acts 2:2 ESV

Believers and nonbelievers alike cannot see the wind, but all can feel and hear the wind.

What winds are you waiting for God to release in your life?

Dear God, Your moves are mighty like the wind. Felt by all. Exposing Your power. Your wonder. Help us to lean into Your wind. Your calling. Your move. Lord, please prepare me for Your wind. I want to be ready for a move of Your wind to fulfill Your many promises. There has been much shaking in my life, which I believe was training wheels for the winds You are preparing me for. With open eyes and a beating heart, I look forward to feeling You blow the winds in directions that take me to heights beyond my wildest dreams. I am looking forward to this wind, *MY WIND*.

Fire and hail, snow and mist, stormy
wind fulfilling his word!

Psalm 148:8 ESV

DO YOU SEE THE LIGHT?

My sweet daughter,
do you see all the good around you?
Do you see the many blessings?
Can you taste your cup of coffee?
Can you feel My presence with you?
Can you see the beauty outside your window?
Do you understand the little blessings
placed in each day?
The small things, some days,
will be the big things

The world and its desires pass away, but whoever
does the will of God lives forever.

John 2:17 NIV

Today I just want you to know
how loved you are by Me, your Creator
How precious your life is to Me
How much I want to fill it with all that is good
Fill it with many blessings, much truth,
lots of beauty, and light

Sometimes all you have to do is sit with
God to experience true peace.

Dear Lord, I pray for more holy moments to fill our everyday lives. More holy moments with just You, Father. 🩶 Do You see what I see, Lord? No, You see much more than I see. So why is it so hard for me to trust You Who sees all things? All I know is, even when I fail to trust, the times I can come and sit with You, I am relieved of all that is weighing heavy on me. I believe this is something only You can do because You are eternal and You make all things beautiful in Your time. You use all things for our good, and because of this, I see the light with You. And I pray that others experience this too. May more souls look to one another and ask, *"DO YOU SEE THE LIGHT?"*

He has made everything beautiful in its time. He has also
set eternity in the human heart; yet no one can fathom
what God has done from beginning to end.

Ecclesiastes 3:11 NIV

MY GARDEN

God created a paradise, a lush garden for us to live in. One where we did not have to work for our food or wear clothes because our minds, our hearts, our eyes were so innocent.

> And he said, "Who told you that you were naked?
> Have you eaten from the tree that I commanded
> you not to eat from?"

Genesis 3:11 NIV

Can you imagine how innocent God created us to be? Man and woman were naked in a garden together and didn't even know it.

This speaks to the way God designed us to live with others. Seeing their naked truths, thoughts, and parts of them and still choosing to believe the best in them and for them. Free of shame and condemnation.

How do I view others when I see their nakedness?

Dear God, restore my vision to an innocent one, like Adam and Eve in the garden. Help me see others through a pure lens—not a measure of good and evil, but of pure love. This world has a way of tainting everything! It teaches us to look for things in others that are not of Your design. Things like racism, classism, and other prejudices hurt both Your heart and human beings. God, I pray for a heart that is pure from the tainted ways of this world. Create a sacred space, a pure garden to live and love. Not one free of problems, but rather filled with understanding that makes it problem-free. May You create a life that reflects Your garden; may You always tend to *MY GARDEN.*

Then the eyes of both of them were opened, and they realized they were naked; so they sewed fig leaves together and made coverings for themselves.

Genesis 3:7 NIV

HOLD YOU

I'm always here to hold you
I'm always here to speak to you
I'm always here to guide you

You shall increase my greatness, And
comfort me on every side.

Psalm 71:21 NKJV

I'm placing longings on your heart
that were not there before
Because there is a time for everything
I'm allowing them to rise
because I am preparing you

If we allow, God will hold us close.
His holding brings relief.

When God holds us close, when we allow Him to, when we invite
Him in, He grows our hearts for a deep yearning. Our Creator shows
us what love looks like. What truth looks like.
God embodies comfort for our minds and souls.

Comfort: The easing or alleviation of a person's feelings
of grief or distress; a state of physical ease and freedom
from pain or constraint.

This comfort follows us and keeps our paths straight. It keeps us going in the direction He has created for our lives. It keeps us on the path that leads to more love, more hope, more peace, and more joy.

Dear God, thank You for all the comfort You have given me through Your love. I experience this comfort when I spend time alone with You and when my eyes are open to the many blessings in my life. I pray for more comforted hearts. 🤍 More hearts to know Your love. God, I invite You in today because I am extra lonely. Rather than turning to a source to hold me that does not feed me, I ask to *HOLD YOU.*

May our Lord Jesus Christ himself and God our Father, who
loved us and by his grace gave us eternal encouragement
and good hope, encourage your hearts and strengthen you
in every good deed and word.

2 Thessalonians 2:16-17 NIV

YOUR STEPS

I am lining up your steps
You will begin to see each one is divine,
each one points to Me

Commit your work to the LORD, and your plans
will be established.

Proverbs 16:3 ESV

I have seen your exhaustion,
I know there have been many moments
filled with discouragement
But I was always there with you,
and I am so proud of you for choosing Me
Please just continue to choose Me
and I will do the rest

He will show you what it looks like
to choose Him.

Commit your way to the LORD; trust in him,
and he will act.

Psalm 37:5 ESV

Before you speak
∽Pray to Me∽

Before you move
∽Pray to Me∽

Before you sleep
∽Pray to Me∽

When you wake
∽Pray to Me∽

When you doubt
∽Pray to Me∽

When you are angry
∽Pray to Me∽

When you are sad
∽Pray to Me∽

When you are happy
∽Pray to Me∽

When you are confused
∽Pray to Me∽

Thus says the LORD, your Redeemer, the Holy One of Israel: "I am the LORD your God, who teaches you to profit, who leads you in the way you should go."

Isaiah 48:17 ESV

My sweet daughter,
all you must do is lay it at My feet
and pray to Me
When you do this, I can do my part
I will direct your steps
and lead the way with ease
With a light
With joy
With patience
With kindness
I direct your steps

Dear Lord, thank You for guiding me this far. I am growing stronger. I can feel it in my every step because I have learned to pray to You before I move! I have desires and needs that feel very far away from me, and on certain days I feel like they are scorching me . . . but You make my bones strong, and with You I will not fail. You make me a well-watered garden, like a spring of flowing water. Kindness and Your Spirit are making the way. Please continue to keep me waiting, looking, and turning to You. I will wait for directions on *YOUR STEPS.*

And the LORD will guide you continually and satisfy your desire in scorched places and make your bones strong; and you shall be like a watered garden, like a spring of water, whose waters do not fail.

Isaiah 58:11 ESV

NOT TO WORRY

My lovely child,
worry is not welcomed in your life
It should not come close to you
I am moving, I am working
on your behalf at all times
I can see worry fade from your life
as you grow closer to Me
It will not and does not
have power over you,
My sweet daughter
This makes Me smile

What makes God smile?

When we are worry free, God smiles.

My sweet child,
whenever you start to worry,
remind yourself this is not from Me,
your Creator 🩶

As you work today,
find something that reminds you
how close I am
Keep your window open
and don't forget to look up
and see Me in the trees

and feel Me in the breeze
Play a song 🎵 that brings Me close,
calms you, excites you, and comforts you
And know how much I love you

Dear God, make me perfect in Your love. Not that I am free from flaws, but the flaws do not consume me. Lack of love in a space allows fear to sneak in, so please protect me with Your love in spaces where there is a lack. Your perfect love protects me, it teaches me *NOT TO WORRY.*

There is no fear in love. But perfect love drives out fear, because fear has to do with punishment. The one who fears is not made perfect in love.

1 John 4:18 NIV

POWER OF TRUTH

I wish you could see all I do
I wish I could pull back the curtains,
My sweet daughter, and
reveal the powerful work
in your life

Why, Lord?

If you could see all I do,
you would understand
the power of and in your precious life
If you could see Me working
on your behalf daily,
you would know what little authority
these negative emotions have,
what little power the lies have
My children would find themselves
in a continuous state of rest if they could see this
I want My children to have ease and rest
I want them to understand what this looks
and feels like in all different seasons
of their lives
No matter the weather

When you are confused, sad, or
hurt, just go to God first.

Ask Me
Seek Me
And I will guide You

Dear Lord, I desire to live in a world filled with more
truth and knowledge of truth because it creates a safe place for
innocent lives, like my little nieces. If there were more souls who
chose Your truth, the kids and little ones would be left alone; they
would grow and not be weighed down by worry or fear because
we'd live in a world removed from all that steals and kills hope,
light, joy, and love! Oh, I know this is the
POWER OF TRUTH.

Who desires all people to be saved and
to come to the knowledge of the truth.

1 Timothy 2:4 ESV

BEAUTY IN TIME

He heals the brokenhearted and binds up their wounds.

Psalm 147:3 ESV

Lord, You have filled my life with so much beauty.
So much goodness. So much love. 🤍

🔑 With time, comes healing and beauty.

Lord, this morning I look out and can feel You in the beauty I see.
I am filled with joy because I have dreams and hopes for a future.
I am filled because I know how powerful and divine Your ways are.
I have seen them work in my life.

Lord, I have not always felt this when I wake in the morning, but
today I do. I'm so grateful for You opening my eyes. I'm so grateful
for the pain and the loss. For the dark days. Because through them,
You have enlightened me.

Dear Lord, thank You for helping me see the beauty in today. 🌷 I
pray more beauty fills the minds of people everywhere. Where Your
beauty is, there is comfort. There is comfort in all You create. Thank
You for planting eternity in our hearts and bringing
BEAUTY IN TIME.

He has made everything beautiful in its time. Also, he has put eternity
into man's heart, yet so that he cannot find out what God has done from
the beginning to the end.

Ecclesiastes 3:11 ESV

MY COLORS

Look at the way I paint this earth
Do you see how the leaves change colors?
How beautiful they are through each season
The bright green, the golden yellow, the fiery purple,
the orange mixed with the blood red,
and the crisp brown
My creation is beautiful and filled with color
My people are beautiful and filled with color
I love all My creation
I smile down on My beautiful creation
I wish My creation would let Me hold them more
I wish they would let Me be with them
through all the seasons
All the changes
All the colors

When you can see the beauty in each
color, know it is from Him.

Seeing the beauty in each color grants freedom.

Seeing the beauty in each color gives life and brings joy.

A thankful heart opens eyes to see.

⦿ 11.22.18 ⦿

Dear Lord, this is the season my sweet father who is now in heaven left this earth. Thanksgiving is a day that will forever be marked. And as I look up, what I see is beauty in Your leaves. So much beauty in Your creation. This brings much comfort to my heart because I was not always able to experience this beauty. I am reminded there is a season for everything. The pain does not last, and with You, there is beauty and blessings in all things. 🤍

🍃 Dear Lord, I pray for more eyes to be opened to see the beauty in pain because we have a choice to live close to You 🙏, and with You, the suffering in life brings more color. As I open my eyes today, I love all I see. I love

MY COLORS.

He will wipe every tear from their eyes. There will be no
more death or mourning or crying or pain, for the old order
of things has passed away.

Revelation 21:4 NIV

DECEMBER

✦ *TRUST* ✦

The majority of your distress
stems from your lack of trust
Have I not always made it clear to you,
My sweet one?
Do I not give you visions
and fill you with hope?

Humble yourselves, therefore, under the mighty hand of
God so that at the proper time he may exalt you, casting
all your anxieties on him, because he cares for you.

1 Peter 5:6-7 ESV

Why, Lord, is it so hard for me to trust? You have been
so good to me.

Because, My sweet daughter,
you place your trust in things that are not Me
You place your trust in what you can see
You place your trust in people
I am your God,
My timing is holy,
and only I want what is best for you
In a way like no other

How do I trust You each day?

You pray to Me
You ask Me
You come to Me
You spend time with Me
so My words can comfort you
Not others' words, but Mine
My trust encourages
Who wants to bless you more than Me?
Your divine Creator

My sweet daughter,
when you trust Me,
you allow Me to move in your life
and on your behalf
Please just continue to honor
all I have currently blessed you with

Trust God. He will guide you. He is never late.

I want you to have joy each day . . .
in the big and little things

Tomorrow will always be there. Yesterday won't.

Dear Lord, You will not delay. The time will pass, so help
us to wait for the vision and the appointed time. It will only be in a
matter of time with You! Help me wait for You, and grow me as I
wait. Use me as I wait. Teach me as I wait. Help us see the training
taking place by Your hand when we face pain. Help us see and
believe in Your mystery, Your magical ways that never bring shame,
but fill us and those we love with more love and truth. My God, the
vision awaits. You will not delay, so today I choose You, for that is
where I place my

TRUST!

For still the vision awaits its appointed time; it hastens to
the end—it will not lie. If it seems slow, wait for it; it
will surely come; it will not delay.

Habakkuk 2:3 ESV

SIMPLE JOYS

The way the lights flicker on the tree and the smile on the snowman's face.

The smell of a Christmas tree 🎄 and my warm morning cup of tea. 🍵

When we are faithful over and with a little, He will set us up with much. So don't wait—run to the Lord and enter into His joy!

Dear Lord, thank You for this morning and the simple joys. Some days I can see the simple joys and they feel like the big ones. In this season, I want to be able to see You and feel You all around me. When this happens, I am comforted. Thank You for allowing a safe and restful home for me to work and live. I have so much to be grateful for in this holiday season. I can't imagine a life without You. I pray for all the people that do not know You. Their eyes are closed to Your joy. Please, I pray for more souls to have Your joy, for more souls to experience the *SIMPLE JOYS.*

His master said to him, "Well done, good and faithful servant. You have been faithful over a little; I will set you over much. Enter into the joy of your master."

Matthew 25:21 ESV

Coming Soon

LOVE LETTERS TO GOD

by Vendela Raquel

*The following pages contain a sneak peek of my forthcoming book,
Love Letters to God, which feature poems that express the ways
God has warmed my heart with both simple and large joys.*

NEW WINE

The need to believe
The need to let go of the disbelief in order to taste the
New wine that flows
Now is the time, ripe and ready
Through the crushing and the pressing
Came new vines, time to drink and enjoy
The labor under the sun that flows from the new skins within
A gift from
You
I can now see, by death my cup was tipped...that was it
A season filled with restless nights, weary mornings and sleepy days
It was there
You met me and now I know the necessity of the
New wine
That flows from within
Time to drink, time to enjoy the cup
You have prepared for Me
So erase my disbelief, lower my walls and let in the love
You wish to stay, let it fill my life as I look to
You
I wake with open eyes and a heart that desires
Truth for
You and all
You do
The signs are there as
You wake me with each rising sun, I am greeted by
Your love
Your joy is planted in me
I have the power to live free
Now that my greatest care is to dwell close to
You
I will experience wonders that could only be from
You
The Creator of all, the Almighty
Truly there is nothing
You can't do
2.25.21 for today marks a season and time filled with
New Wine

FORGIVE

Innocent and pure
Yet unforgiveness dwells close
Thick and strong the chains
Around my heart will grow
If I don't
Let go
Help me place it all in
Your hands

Please, show me how to hand it over to
You
I know unforgiveness blocks love
Please, help me
Let go

Why do I doubt…
Is it not
You who has always taken care of me?
You who has always comforted me?
You who has always made a way?
You who has always lifted me high
And made all things right?

You will be my reason to forgive
You are enough
Your promises are enough
Your love is enough
Please help me
Forgive

SEE LIKE YOU

I see odds
I see risk
I see greener grass on the other side
I see grand mountains
Help me to trust
Help me to
See like
You
You see the beginning and the end
You see the path
You see the how
You see the possibilities
My thoughts so limited
My ways lack much faith
Oh how I long
I need to see like
You
As
You prepare to do
What only
You can do
Make the impossible possible
Help me to trust
Help me to
See Like You

Not by might nor by power, but by my Spirit
—Lord Almighty—

Zechariah 4:6 NIV